PRAIS
LAWYER WELLNESS I

"*Lawyer Wellness is Not an Oxymoron* has the potential to not only save individual lawyers from living a dissatisfying life, but to restore life back into our weathered profession, and in turn secure its future. This is a book to be lived by all lawyers."

Danielle Rondeau
Killam Cordell Murray
Founder of *Trash Your Stress*, Vancouver

"Andy Clark underscores the critically important reality, which he supports with overwhelming evidence, that lawyers are not a happy and healthy group of professionals. He states emphatically that there is a solution and then offers a detailed roadmap for achieving these goals."

Bob Barasa
Attorney and CEO, Barasa Consulting, LLC, Chicago

"*Lawyer Wellness Is Not an Oxymoron*, but it is an essential tool for achieving health, happiness and fulfillment. It is the Bluebook for getting the most out of your life and your practice."

Brian Early
Early, Lucarelli, Sweeney & Strauss, New York

"With the stress of practicing law and having a successful law practice in today's legal environment, plus wanting to "have it all"—being greedy enough to think you can achieve that success plus be happy, healthy and fulfilled in all aspects of your life—if this is you, then you need to STOP in your tracks, take a step back and learn from Andy's exceptional insights. I truly wish the book had been available 25+ years ago when I started my own law practice and wonder now what I would have done differently."

Jean Einstein
Einstein Law Ltd., Chicago

"Andy Clark is the 'Wealthy Barber of Wellness'! I have read several books offering wisdom and self-help that were nowhere near as enjoyable and readable as his. I also do not think his advice and approach is limited—or should be limited—to lawyers; it works for any professional—or any busy person for that matter. He inspired me to start taking the stairs."

Hugh Cameron
Stewart McKelvey, Fredericton, NB

"*Lawyer Wellness is Not an Oxymoron* is a much needed read. This book takes an in-depth look at the way lawyers think and the factors that drive and motivate attorneys. It is a positive reminder to lawyers that taking care of themselves is taking care of the bottom line. Lawyer Wellness translates into higher profits, greater recognition and advanced achievement. I applaud Andy Clark for his efforts to advance and to improve the profession.

Gloria Legette
Attorney, Chicago

"This book is a brilliant deep dive into the truth behind what it takes to have an extraordinary life in the legal world. Clark gives it to you raw and uncut, sharing his own intimate personal experiences, and taking you into your future where your commitment to personal wellness produces career success AND a healthy, happy, and fulfilling life. If you've secretly realized that your current formula for success as an attorney might not be all it's cracked up to be…if you dream of a more enriching career with your vitality intact…then Lawyer Wellness is Not an Oxymoron holds the keys to your satisfaction and is a must read.

Damion S. Lupo
Author of *Reinvented Life*, Austin, TX

LAWYER WELLNESS IS NOT AN OXYMORON

WHY TOMORROW'S TOP LAWYERS MUST
EMBRACE WELLNESS TODAY—
AND WHAT YOU NEED TO DO TO BE ONE OF THEM

ANDY CLARK

Lawyer Wellness is Not an Oxymoron

Copyright © 2013 by Andy Clark.

Inquiries should be addressed to:

Andy Clark
30 Hughes St.
Fredericton, NB, Canada
E3A 2W3

www.wellnesslawyer.com

First Edition
First Printing November 2013

Cover design by: Elizabeth Novak
Layout by: Jake Muelle
Author's photograph by: Heather Grattan

ISBN 978-0-9921574-0-1 print
ISBN 978-0-9921574-1-8 electronic

1. Law Practice 2. Health & Fitness 3. Wellness & Quality of Life

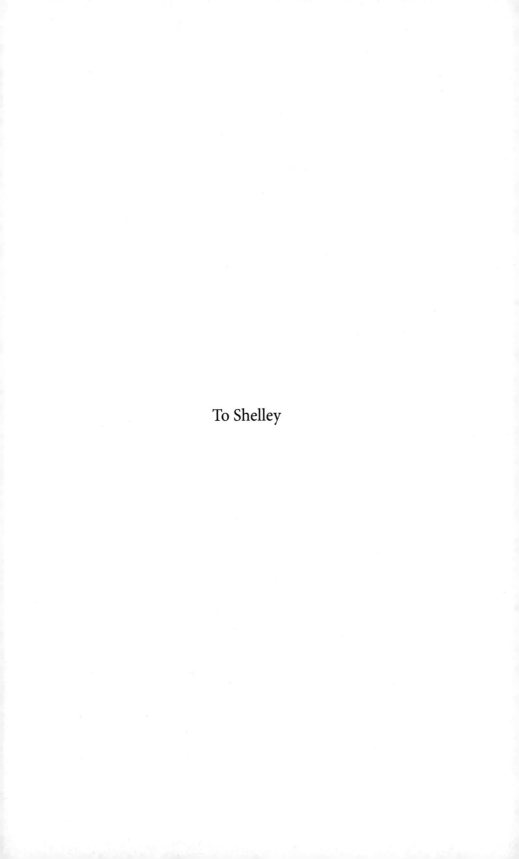

To Shelley

"When health is absent, wisdom cannot reveal itself, art cannot manifest, strength cannot fight, wealth becomes useless, and intelligence cannot be applied."

—Herophilus

CONTENTS

INTRODUCTION

WHAT THIS BOOK IS ABOUT

A couple of years ago, I presented a lecture at a Canadian provincial bar association conference. Prior to my presentation there was a luncheon during which one of the lawyers at my table asked me where I practiced. I told him that I no longer practiced law full-time, that I had become a wellness entrepreneur, and I was going to be speaking after lunch on the topic of lawyer wellness. The lawyer looked at me curiously, paused for a moment, and then said "Well, that's the secret to lawyer wellness...stop practicing law!" He laughed, I laughed, and the rest of the table had a good laugh, too.

As part of an ice-breaking conversation at a legal conference, the lawyer's comment was funny. But the broader implication of his remark was not. It represents the view of many lawyers that the term *lawyer wellness* is an oxymoron; that it is not possible to be well and to live well while practicing law.

Why is it that so many lawyers believe that sacrificing personal wellness is part of the price of admission to practice law? And, perhaps more importantly, why are so many lawyers prepared to pay that lofty price?

Including law school, my life in law has now spanned over 15 years. In that time, I have seen far too many lawyer friends and colleagues struggle under the weight of their personal and professional responsibilities. Evidence abounds that the same rings true across the profession. Thousands of lawyers throughout the world suffer from one or more of the 3 Uns: They are unhappy, unhealthy, or unfulfilled. Many lawyers experience two of the 3 Uns on a sustained basis. Some experience all three.

Despite what many in our profession believe, none of the 3 Uns is a necessary requirement of practicing law—we just make excuses and let them be. Lawyers are *not* martyrs. Self-sacrifice is *not* a necessary component of the job description. While each of the 3 Uns will undoubtedly show up in your career and in the rest of your life from time to time, the fact is that life is too short and your role as a lawyer is too important for you to experience any of the 3 Uns on a chronic basis. When any of the 3 Uns show up as perpetual pain in your life, not only do *you* suffer, but your *family and loved ones* suffer right along with you. And from a professional perspective, when lawyers suffer in this manner, their career and clients suffer too, as does the profession itself.

As this book will demonstrate, the 3 Uns are the *effects* of failing to live a wellness lifestyle. In other words, you cannot achieve sustained health, happiness, and fulfillment without embracing and adopting wellness in your life on a daily basis. You might be able to achieve sporadic health, happiness, and fulfillment, but without living a wellness lifestyle it is impossible to experience all three on a sustained basis. This book will show you why.

Of course, in order to demonstrate that a wellness lifestyle is the blueprint for sustained health, happiness, and fulfillment as a lawyer, I'll have to define what, exactly, I mean by a wellness lifestyle. Actually, I'll need to back up a step further and define what the heck *wellness* means, since it has become such an over-used and misused term in recent years. Many lawyers (and law firms) think they know what wellness is, and they believe that the steps they are taking to implement so-called wellness into their lives (or workplaces) are sufficient. Most of them are wrong.

By reading this book, you'll discover once and for all what real wellness is and what it means to live a wellness lifestyle. More than that, you will learn *why* you need to embrace and adopt a wellness lifestyle, and you will learn *how* to do it, too. You will discover that now more than ever, as the legal services landscape moves away from the "work longer" or "time and effort" business model and towards a more results-oriented model based on innovation and effectiveness, lawyers who don't adopt a wellness lifestyle today will do so at their peril. Now more than ever, lawyers who don't invest in their personal wellness put themselves at a competitive disadvantage in their legal career—not to mention in their lives as a whole. Simply put, lawyers who do not adopt a wellness lifestyle today will fall further behind in the coming years as the legal services business rapidly evolves. This book will show you why this is so—and it will give you the information, ideas, and resources you need to make sure you can thrive in tomorrow's legal services landscape; to make sure you're not one of the lawyers left behind.

I should also make clear at the outset what this book is *not* about. With all the mixed messages that abound about wellness these days, you can be forgiven for thinking that "wellness lawyers" spend all day practicing yoga, juicing (the good kind of juicing), meditating, volunteering at the Boys and Girls Club, and, in their spare time, cranking out a few billable hours—on "save the world" files. Nope, this book is not about being home at five o'clock every night for dinner with the kids; it's not about exercising three hours a day or never eating chocolate cake again; and it's certainly not about forsaking your responsibilities to your clients, your firm, and the profession while you put out a positive vibe to the universe and wait for the law of attraction to come to your rescue. On the contrary, this book will show you very logically and very practically how living a wellness lifestyle allows you to bring more to the party in all aspects of your life. It will show you that it's possible to create an extraordinary law career within an extraordinary life—not at the expense of one.

WHO SHOULD READ THIS BOOK

This book was primarily written for lawyers, obviously, and I think all lawyers will benefit from reading it. I expect that it will benefit you most if:

> ➤ You're a lawyer who regularly experiences one or more of the 3 Uns
> ➤ You're a lawyer who isn't as healthy, happy, or fulfilled as you would like to be

> ➤ You're a lawyer who wants to become more effective and to gain a competitive advantage in tomorrow's legal services landscape
> ➤ You're a law student or you're considering a career in law

The book was not written for lawyers who know they're on their way out of practice—there are plenty of career counseling and "transition out of law" books out there for that. It's more for lawyers who intend to find a way to practice law in a manner that enhances, rather than erodes, their overall quality of life.

If you're not a lawyer, you don't plan to become one, and you've happened to pick up this book, you'll find it useful too. A lot of the information provided and principles presented can be applied by anyone wanting to increase their degree of wellness and quality of life. And, of course, once you're done with it, you can leave your copy at your lawyer's office the next time you drop in!

WHY THIS BOOK WAS WRITTEN

Despite the litany of lawyer jokes on the theme of our gruesome death and/or mass extermination[1], we're kind of a big deal in this world. Lawyers are essential to the proper and orderly functioning of society. So we can't all quit, right? Fortunately, none of us have to. Notwithstanding the view of my new, wisecracking conference delegate friend, quitting practice is not the secret to wellness. Lawyer wellness is not an oxymoron. You can have a great law practice *and* a high degree of wellness in your life. This book was written to show lawyers not only that it is possible to do so, but that it is incumbent upon us to do so.

Our increasingly complex society requires ever-increasingly complex laws to ensure the rule of law, and it's not your Average Joe or Jane who can make sense of those laws and provide guidance to those who don't. Lawyers' skills are varied and many, but chief among them is intelligence. There may be some bad lawyers in the world, but there are not too many dumb ones. You need a high level of smarts to do this job.

Yet for all of our collective intelligence, we don't, as a group, live our lives all that intelligently. If, as Ralph Waldo Emerson said, "the first wealth is health"; if, as Aristotle said, "happiness is the meaning and purpose of life"; and if, as Abraham Maslow said, "what human beings can be, they must be"; why do so many of us fail to achieve sustained health, happiness, and fulfillment? This is the Great Lawyer Riddle—and this book was written to help you solve it.

This book was written to show you that it is time to take charge of your level of health, happiness, and fulfillment. It was written to urge you to stop blaming your firm, the business model, or the profession when one or more of the 3 Uns show up in your life. It was written to demonstrate that your degree of wellness has the single biggest influence over your quality of life, and that it is primarily under your control.

I am not the first person to examine the issue of wellness (or lack thereof) in our profession. There are 1.2 million lawyers in the United States. There's another million in India, and another 300,000 or so in the United Kingdom, Canada, Australia, and New Zealand. That's 2.5 million lawyers, and they are just a portion of all of the lawyers in the world. Of course, many lawyers *have* figured out a way to thrive personally and professionally. But, as we'll see in this book, a significant percentage experience one or more of the 3 Uns in their career and overall lives. That translates into hundreds of thousands of lawyers who aren't fully healthy, happy and fulfilled, and that's a problem.

Thankfully, many people before me have recognized this. There are several books and articles about various aspects of lawyers' wellbeing written by lawyers and non-lawyers alike. I reference some of them in this book. A recent study commissioned by the Canadian Bar Association examined the issue[2], and at the time of writing, a similar study is being conducted in Australia.[3] In the United States, the American Bar Association has spearheaded several conferences, studies, and projects over the last two decades aimed at tackling lawyers' health, happiness, and quality of life issues[4], and at least one American law school offers a course on the subject.[5] Most, if not all, major state and provincial bar associations have recognized the obstacles that practicing law presents when it comes to the wellbeing of its practitioners, and consequently have set up lawyer assistance programs to help their members who struggle with physical, mental, or emotional health issues. All of these books, articles, studies, and programs are helpful. But they're not enough.

With this book I hope to contribute to the lawyer wellness discussion by bringing some new perspectives to it. The purpose of the book isn't to change the profession from the top down; rather it is to empower individual lawyers to understand how they can—and why they must—help themselves become more effective lawyers and live healthier, happier, more fulfilling lives. The health of the profession is intricately tied to the health of its lawyers. If lawyers are healthier, the profession will be healthier. It's as simple as that.

And yet, in some cases it's not as simple as that, because there is a larger health crisis to consider that extends beyond the profession. Rates of chronic illness (obesity, diabetes, heart disease, cancer, and so on) have reached epidemic proportions in modern society. There are many contributing factors for this, but chief among them is the illogical paradigm in which much of modern health care is delivered. Lawyers are uniquely positioned to challenge this paradigm and to become leaders in the war on chronic illness. In this respect, lawyers have a role to play that is larger than many realize.

Just think, if lawyers—the absolute *last* group of people that most others would associate with high levels of wellness—became the healthiest professionals in our society, that would positively and profoundly change the world. This book was written to inspire lawyers everywhere to rise to that challenge.

1

WHY YOU NEED TO CARE
ABOUT WELLNESS—TODAY

In the chapters that follow, this book will tell you exactly how living a wellness lifestyle creates sustained health, happiness, and fulfillment, and it will tell you what you need to know and do in order to live a wellness lifestyle. So the rest of the book is mostly about the *how*. This first chapter is all about the *why*. As in, *why should I care about wellness and living a wellness lifestyle anyway?* And, *what's in it for me if I do?*

I dig into the concepts of health, happiness, and fulfillment more completely in the next chapter, but I'm going to assume for now that you have a general sense of what each of these things are and that you agree that these are each worthy goals to pursue— that life is better when you are healthy, happy, and fulfilled.

As for what constitutes wellness and living a wellness lifestyle, those concepts are covered in depth in Chapter 3. For now, just know that wellness is defined as "the degree to which an individual experiences health and vitality in any dimension of life," and lifestyle is defined as "a manner of living." A wellness lifestyle, therefore, is "a manner of living that enhances the degree to which you experience health and vitality in your life."

Wellness is much more than just eating right and exercising. Those things are very important, of course, but wellness is really about expressing health and vitality across the whole spectrum of your life: physically, mentally, socially, emotionally, professionally, financially, spiritually, and the list goes on. (The different dimensions of life are explored more fully in Chapter 4.) This is because when you experience stress in *any* area of your life, it creates stress in *every* area of your life. In other words, you need to function at a high level in every important area of your life in order to avoid chronic negative stress from showing up everywhere in your life. This may appear to be a daunting—even impossible—task, but I assure you it is not. In the chapters that follow, the book will show you how to achieve this.

THE GREAT LAWYER RIDDLE

Since you're a lawyer, you are smart enough to know that wellness and taking care of yourself are important things. And if you're like the vast majority of lawyers, you're not living under the poverty line. Therefore, if you experience one or more of the 3 Uns—unhealthy, unhappy, unfulfilled—on a sustained basis, then neither your ignorance nor socio-economic status reasonably can be put forth as the reason why.

So the Great Lawyer Riddle is this: If we're so smart, how come so many of us are not as healthy, happy, and fulfilled as we'd like to be?

The easy answer is to blame the nature of the practice and the prevailing business model. To be sure, there isn't much in the nature of law practice that promotes a whole lot of wellness. Demanding clients, tight deadlines, and billing pressures combine to create little free time and lots of stress. Your work can be the difference between your client gaining or losing significant sums of money, gaining or losing access to their children, gaining or losing their freedom—and in some jurisdictions, gaining or losing their *life*. It doesn't get much more high-stakes than that. That's the nature of the practice. That's what we signed up for.

As a result, many lawyers assume that the 3 Uns are a necessary, unavoidable side effect of practicing law. *It's just part of the package*, they say. *It's the price of admission to the practice of law.* They're not thrilled about it, but *that's just the way it is.* Some lawyers even wear these side effects as a perverse badge of honor, bragging that they haven't slept in three days or haven't taken a vacation in five years, as if that makes them more of a "real lawyer" (whatever that means). These lawyers likely consider themselves to be *realists*. But, as lawyer stress management expert and author Amiram Elwork, Ph.D., argues, such an approach is misguided. He writes, "I do not believe that passive endurance of chronic stress is a sign of courage or character. Because chronic stress is so harmful to your physical and mental health, simply enduring it is generally a sign of bad judgment. Overcoming life's challenges, not just enduring them, is what takes real guts and ingenuity."[6]

Yes, practicing law is among the world's most demanding professions. Yes, lawyering can be a tough—a *really* tough—gig. But does that mean we must always put client demands and necessities ahead of our own? Does that mean we must *ever* put client demands and necessities ahead of our own?

As lawyers, part of our job is to take responsibility for our clients' issues and to help them achieve a desired result. But so few of us take responsibility over our own lives to ensure we achieve *our* desired result—and part of the reason is that many of us don't know what our desired result is. Lawyers may be an intelligent bunch when it comes to analyzing the law and advising clients on how to best comply with it. But if, as entrepreneur and quality of life expert Jon Butcher has said, "true intelligence is measured by how intelligently you live your life", then we're nowhere near the head of the class.

A big part of the reason for this is that we don't take the time to figure out *how* to live more intelligently. The number one reason why so many lawyers go through much of their careers and their lives experiencing one or more of the 3 Uns is that they never take the time to seriously contemplate what *would* make them healthy and happy and fulfilled. They never turn their minds to the issue of figuring out exactly what their ideal life— full of health, happiness, and fulfillment—looks like. Or, as one legal scholar put it: "Lawyers don't sit down and think logically about why they are leading the lives they are leading any more than buffalo sit down and think logically about why they are stampeding."[7]

In our day job, we often craft arguments about who's at fault in a given fact pattern, but arguing that others are at fault when we experience one or more of the 3 Uns isn't going to win us the case. It's not the responsibility of your clients nor the profession to make sure you are healthy, happy, and fulfilled. Your firm or employer certainly can play a supporting role to help out—it's in their best interest to do so—but it's not their job either. Ultimately, the level of your health, happiness, and fulfillment is up to you. You, and only you, are responsible for it. You weren't genetically programmed to be unhealthy, unhappy, or unfulfilled. You didn't relinquish your rights to experience health, happiness, and fulfillment when you were admitted to practice. If you're unhealthy, unhappy, or unfulfilled and you are waiting for your clients to stop bothering you (while still happily paying you), or if you're waiting for your firm to pay for your gym membership *and* to check in with you every day to make sure you actually use it, or if you're waiting for the profession to place lawyers' personal wellness at the top of its priority list…well, you'll be doing an awful lot of waiting.

In this respect, many lawyers are falling down on the job. They aren't taking responsibility for their wellness, and therefore they continue to experience one or more of the 3 Uns on a sustained basis. That impacts their quality of life and, importantly, the quality of life of their loved ones, too. Lawyers intuitively know this, yet most often it's not enough to compel them to embrace and embark upon a course of action that will yield more health, happiness, and fulfillment. I'm not necessarily talking about a career change or any other form of total life overhaul here. That may be required in some cases, but that will be the exception. I'm talking about getting conscious about *why* you are leading the life you are leading, and about what causes in your life have created the *effect* of poor health, unhappiness, or lack of fulfillment. I'm talking about understanding how the sum total of your past choices and actions across the whole spectrum of your life add up to the quality of life you are leading now. I'm talking about creating some new habits and replacing some old ones that, over time, will yield improved and lasting health. I'm talking about adopting a wellness lifestyle.

WELLNESS: WHAT'S IN IT FOR ME?

Just because wellness is a buzzword these days doesn't mean it should automatically be something you should care about. If adopting a wellness lifestyle is going to be more effort than it's worth to you, then what's the point, right? So if you're asking yourself, *Wellness…what's in it for me?* you're asking the right question. It's essential to get clear on the benefits of adopting a wellness lifestyle before you invest the time, energy, and resources to do so.

When I speak to non-lawyers about this, I focus on demonstrating that living a wellness lifestyle is so important because your level of wellness is the single biggest factor influencing your health, happiness, and fulfillment—three things that are major determinants of the quantity and quality of your life. If having a long life full of health, happiness, and fulfillment is important to you, then a focus on wellness now—today—is a prerequisite.

I ask people to spend some time considering this. Are quantity and quality of life important to you? They're not to everybody. Some people want quantity, but they don't necessarily care about increasing quality; their lives are okay, and they're okay with just being okay for the rest of their lives. They tend to sacrifice the present for the future. On the other hand, some people don't give a hoot about quantity—how long they live—but boy do they ever want quality! These are the people who go as hard as they can for as long as they can, knowing it might not be that long in the end. These people will have some pretty great times and great experiences, but more than likely their life will be cut short. They sacrifice the future for the now.

The vast majority of people, however, value both quantity *and* quality of life. To these people I say that living a wellness lifestyle is the only way for you to achieve that goal. I tell them that the single most important thing you will ever learn about wellness is this: Wellness is a means to an end, and the end is quantity and quality of life. Wellness is *not* the end game. You don't seek a higher degree of wellness so you can go around at cocktail parties saying, "See how well I am?" or "I am sooooo well today!" (Well, I suppose you could, but sooner or later you wouldn't find yourself on the invite list for cocktail parties anymore.)

Quantity and Quality of Life

What do quantity and quality of life mean? Quantity is pretty simple: It's how long you live. This is easily measured; it's simply how old you are when you die. Quality, on the other hand, is a little tougher to get a handle on. Quality of life is about how *well* you live. One person's well might be another person's hell, so quality of life is much more subjective and much harder to measure than is quantity. That said, there are not too many lawyers on this planet for whom health, happiness, and fulfillment are not three key ingredients in their quality of life recipe. Yes, there are millions of people in our world who live in poverty, in war-torn countries, or under oppressive political regimes for whom *survival* is the primary (if not only) goal of existence. For those people, health, happiness, and fulfillment may be the stuff of fantasy. But if you're a lawyer reading this book, that probably doesn't apply to you.

You can find some complex definitions of quality of life out there if you look. A Google search on the subject will keep you reading for days. I prefer a simpler definition: *Quality of life is the degree of freedom you enjoy across all dimensions of your life.*

By freedom, I don't mean civil liberties. It's not about comparing life in the industrialized West to life in politically oppressive nations. It's about degrees of freedom among people who live and work alongside each other in free societies.

To explain, let's look at two hypothetical lawyers who have different degrees of freedom, to see who has the higher quality of life.

Meet Bill and Susan. Both are 52-year-old tax lawyers. Both are partners at 100-lawyer firms. Both have recorded an average of 2000 hours and have earned approximately $400,000 in each of the last five years.

Bill plans to begin pulling back on his client commitments over the next year, in order to retire at age 55. He has been smart with his money and he and his family have lived fairly modestly during his working years (if you call a five-bedroom house in a good part of town and two adventure trips a year living modestly).

From a financial perspective, he could retire now, but he enjoys practicing law and the people he works with, so he wants to gradually phase out of practice over a few years. He and his wife Jamie are already planning a trip around the world when he turns 55, and he is really looking forward to that. They are going to bring their three grown children along for a portion of the trip, too—the Peru leg of the journey when they'll be doing a lot of hiking and visiting Machu Picchu, one of Bill's lifelong dreams. Bill will probably do some consulting work in his retirement to keep busy, and to share his expertise with those who need it—but only as long as he wants to and if it doesn't interfere too much with his triathlon training (he wants to finish top-10 at the national over-50 championships) and Jamie's travel plans.

For Susan, the joy of practicing tax law has long since faded. She does it because she makes good money at it, but she's never been able to keep much of it. She wouldn't consider herself a spendthrift, but everything she brings in seems to go out the door just as quickly—sometimes more. Her first husband cited her spending habits as a reason for their divorce. She shares custody of her three kids with him. She has fallen out of love with her second husband, but after the expense of her first divorce, she feels she's better off just sticking it out. She figures she'll have to keep working for a good 10-15 more years in order to have enough money for retirement—if she's able to change her spending habits. And she's worried that some of her chronic health issues—hypertension and Type 2 Diabetes—will keep getting worse and will get more expensive as she ages. She thinks often that it might be time to make use of the fitness membership and other wellness programs her firm offers, but she's just so damn busy. Maybe next month.

Who has more health, financial, career, and relationship freedom: Bill or Susan? Who has a higher quality of life?

Obviously these examples are designed to showcase complete opposite sides of the spectrum with respect to lawyer wellness. But I bet you can think of two lawyers you know who come close to meeting these descriptions. Some lawyers, despite making half a million dollars per year or more, really have little freedom in their lives, and their quality of life suffers as a result.

If you have complete freedom of what, when, where, how and with, then you'll have a great a quality of life. Of course, very few people have *complete* freedom in this respect, but even fewer wouldn't *want* more of it in their lives. And let's get this clear at the outset: Quality of life is *not* dependent on having more money. Money can help improve quality of life in some ways, but it is not the determining factor. As we'll see in the next chapter, money has little do with finding sustained health, happiness, and fulfillment. Your level of wellness is by far more important to your quality of life than money, or any other single factor in your life. The old adage is true: Health=Wealth. Truer still: Wellness=Wealth.

YEAH, WELLNESS IS IMPORTANT, BUT I'LL GET TO IT LATER

All of this is great stuff, right? You're going to run out right now and buy some new runners, a new road bike, and a new speedo and crush that triathlon next month, right? You're going to eat a bunch of kale and chia seeds for supper tonight, have the leftovers for breakfast, and you're going to lose that 15 pounds once and for all, right? You're going to do this, that, and the other thing to embrace wellness so that you give yourself more likelihood of achieving greater quantity and quality of life, right?

Well, if you're like most lawyers, you won't. I hope I'm wrong, but even though everything you've read so far is logical and reasonable and makes good sense, and even though you know that investing more time, energy, and resources in your personal wellness is really something you should do, you won't. You might for a day, or a week, or even a month, but you'll run into some obstacles and you'll end up confirming your self-fulfilling prophecy that there are just too many demands inherent in practicing law to keep up with your wellness lifestyle implementation initiative.

Intuitively, if not consciously, you already knew all of this anyway. You know that eating right, exercising, and managing negative stress in your life are good for you and will dramatically increase your chances of experiencing a long and happy life alongside your loved ones. You know that doing these things consistently will dramatically decrease your chances of leaving behind a widowed spouse and orphaned children, of being the father your daughter cries about at her wedding because you're not there, of being the grandmother your grandkids will never be able to play with. Yet somehow, if you're like most lawyers, that's not enough to compel you to actually do anything about it on a consistent, sustained basis. When you're constantly under the gun to discharge your mountain of daily personal and professional responsibilities, as most lawyers are, there's not much bandwidth left to think about the future, much less plan for it.

In *The Lawyer Bubble: A Profession in Crisis*, Steven Harper writes that, as a result of the prevailing business model in the profession—most prevalent at large law firms—geared towards maximizing billable hours, client billings, and associate-to-partner leverage ratios, lawyers have "become trapped in the culture of short-termism."[8] This short-termism in our career tends to spill over into our personal lives too. Indeed, the shortsightedness in our personal lives may be the *result* of the short-termism in our career: *I've got to get this work done now; I'll get to my health and relationships later.* Often *later* doesn't come—at least not until it's too late.

So if the prospect of improved quantity and quality of life for yourself and your loved ones isn't enough to compel you to adopt a wellness lifestyle, then what is? Well, given that lawyers are generally a pretty competitive bunch, who place a high value on career performance and success, what if I can show you that a wellness lifestyle makes you a better, more effective lawyer? What if you were able to own the fact that when you are well in all dimensions of your life, you give yourself a tremendous competitive advantage in your career? What if it might even help you make more money? Would that get your attention? Would that compel you to act?

And what if you realized that this is true now more than ever, at a time when, as many experts and most observers believe, we're on the precipice of sweeping change in the legal profession? There is, as Steven Harper points out in his book, a lawyer bubble in the profession right now: far too many lawyers and far too few clients willing to pay legal fees based solely on billable hours. Famed author and legal prognosticator Richard Susskind calls this the "more-for-less challenge".[9] More than ever, clients are demanding more value for their legal spend. Increasingly, clients are expecting their lawyers to deliver more results for less money and in less time.

According to Susskind, the "more-for-less" challenge is one of the three major trends in the legal profession that are precipitating its evolution. The second is liberalization of the legal market, which will see (in the jurisdictions that haven't seen it already) non-lawyers permitted to provide legal services. The third is exponentially developing information and communications technologies.

Think about this for a minute. You work hard now. You already practice within an ultra-competitive marketplace. What's going to happen when clients continue to value shop for legal services, not just amongst lawyers, but also amongst corporations and other organizations that are also permitted to bid for and provide legal work? Incidentally, these other entities probably aren't shackled to a billable hour culture and they probably know a lot more about marketing, communications, and client service than most law firms do. And while this is happening, you're expected to be on call 24/7 since the whole world has turned into a virtual office. Do you think these three trends, as they continue to play out in the years ahead, might make the practice of law even *more* competitive? Even *more* stressful? Of course they will.

Who will rise to the top in the new legal landscape? Who will be best positioned to survive and thrive when the lawyer bubble bursts? Those who adopt a wellness lifestyle today—that's who. Because the solution isn't to work harder; it can't be. Most lawyers have little, if any, bandwidth left to work harder. The only solution is to work smarter, to be more effective in the delivery of legal services, and to provide more value for your clients. And as we'll see below, lawyers who experience the benefits of living a wellness lifestyle will be in the best position to do just that.

THE WELLNESS LIFESTYLE ADVANTAGE

We shouldn't need a business reason for wellness, but the reality is that most lawyers are motivated more by business, improving their careers, and gaining more acceptance, reverence, status, and money than they are by being healthy and increasing their chances of living a long, happy, satisfying life.

If you need a business reason for adopting a wellness lifestyle, it is this: Your ability to provide consistent value to your clients, and thus to generate wealth today and in the future, is diminished to the degree to which you are not well in all dimensions of life. Lawyers who *are* well in all dimensions of life are healthier, happier, and more fulfilled *and* they are more effective lawyers. Lawyers who practice law within a wellness lifestyle give themselves a competitive advantage in the legal field, and in life.

Here are just six of the massive career benefits you will experience as a result of living a wellness lifestyle:

> You'll think better
> You'll have more energy
> You'll experience less stress
> You'll gain enhanced confidence
> You'll enjoy a greater sense of control
> You'll develop a clearer sense of purpose

In the chapters that follow, you'll discover the specific ways in which a wellness lifestyle results in each of these benefits for your career. For now, simply consider this: If you could have all of the benefits listed above, without requiring a major life overhaul, would you want them? Do you think they would help you to become a more effective lawyer? And if money is a top value for you, might these benefits allow you to make more of it?

As mentioned above, today's legal landscape is shifting rapidly and permanently. The inefficiencies that were buried in the billable hour model are being unearthed and rejected. Tomorrow's legal services landscape will be built on effectiveness. Tomorrow's lawyers (to borrow the title of Susskind's great book) must be strategic and effective—not just billable hour machines.

What does it mean to be effective? The dictionary says that being effective means producing results, producing favorable impressions, and being ready for action. In practice, being effective requires three things: productivity, efficiency, and achieving meaningful results. Each of these three things is valuable on its own, but you need all three in order to be truly effective.

You can be productive in the sense of generating a lot of work product (i.e. a pile of billable hours), but if it took you twice as long as it should have and the results of your work don't achieve your client's desired results, you haven't been effective. You might have been able to send out a big bill, and the client might even have begrudgingly paid it, but you have not been effective, and your client will probably go elsewhere for their future legal service needs.

You can be efficient in the sense of completing a project in less time and with fewer resources than your competitor. But even though your work product may be of similar or greater quality than your competitor's, it won't be effective unless it achieves meaningful results for your client. As Peter Drucker famously said, "There is nothing so useless as doing efficiently that which should not be done at all."

So to be effective you need the hat trick of productivity, efficiency, and meaningful results. Effectiveness is what clients have begun to demand en masse and what they will continue to demand of their counsel in the future. Most clients don't mind paying for legal services, but they want value for their money. Effective lawyers provide excellent value. Ineffective lawyers do not.

The benefits listed above that result from living a wellness lifestyle will enhance your effectiveness as lawyer significantly. If you consistently think better, and have more energy, confidence, control, and purpose in your life, all while experiencing less stress, you're going to be a much more effective lawyer. Period.

LET'S TALK ABOUT MONEY

Will this put more money in your pocket? It's been a couple of years since I practiced law full-time, but I remember enough to know that it's probably not a good idea for me to guarantee in writing that you're going to make more money. So let me be clear: I am not guaranteeing that you will make more money by adopting a wellness lifestyle. But I think there's a pretty good case for it.

First off, I want to note that most of the literature that I have reviewed on the subject of lawyers and the legal profession has a bias against lawyers who make a ton of money or who help big business make or save a ton of money. Most authors on the subject imply (if they don't say it outright) that there's less nobility in that kind of practice, that it does nothing to help the public good, and that you won't find true happiness or fulfillment there.

I disagree. I think that it's just fine for lawyers to want to make a ton of money, to actually make a ton of money, and to help big business make or save a ton of money. I also think that it's just fine for lawyers *not* to make a ton of money (but to make a comfortable living), and for lawyers to spend their career ensuring that big business doesn't make or save a ton of money at the expense of future generations. As long as a lawyer creates value for the client, serves the client's interests to the best of his or her ability, and does so ethically and within the spirit and intent of his or her professional responsibility obligations, who's to judge what constitutes nobility in the practice of law? As we'll see in a later chapter, making a ton of money won't guarantee health, happiness, and fulfillment, but *not* making a ton of money won't either. Making money—a little or a lot—in a manner that is congruent with your values and interests *will* improve your chances of happiness. As a mentor of mine wisely said, *money simply enhances who you already are.* If you're a good person, making more money will allow you to be more of a good person. If you're a jerk, making more money will allow you to be more of a jerk. So I, for one, am a proponent of removing morality and nobility from the discussion when talking about how much money lawyers make or don't make. There are Big Law partners who make $3 million a year who are wonderful lawyers and wonderful people, and there are Big Law partners who make $3 million a year who are anything but.

What kind of lawyer and person are you? Well, if you use money and love people, you're probably a lawyer I'd like to work with. If you love money and use people, I'm not sure I'd want to spend a whole lot of time with you—or much money on your services.

So how might a wellness lifestyle put more money in your pocket? For starters, let's talk about *longevity*. Lawyers make money when they are working. They don't make money when they are not. If you don't take care of yourself now, health problems will creep into your life earlier rather than later, and when these become serious enough, they will impede your ability to work and to earn income. I'm no math expert, but it seems to me that a lawyer who makes $250,000 a year for 40 years will earn twice as much over a lifetime than a lawyer who makes $250,000 a year for 20 years. If you're 45 years old and you can no longer practice law due to physical or mental health issues, how financially secure will you and your family be in the future? Living a wellness lifestyle today significantly reduces the likelihood that you'll ever have to ask yourself that question.

Second, let's talk about *value*. As mentioned above, tomorrow's lawyers will be paid for the value they create for clients, not for hours worked. Creating more value will require you to be more productive, and efficient, and to achieve more meaningful results, all in less time. Remember Susskind's more-for-less challenge. You'll need to be at the top of your game in order to rise to this challenge. You'll need to think better, have more energy, and reduce distractions. You'll need to minimize professional and non-professional stress, and you'll need to process and dissipate what stress you do experience more quickly. You'll certainly need loads of confidence and to be on purpose every day. These are all benefits you'll experience from living a wellness lifestyle.

Longevity and value creation are on the *making money* side of the equation. What about *keeping money*? That's where a wellness lifestyle can *really* pay financial dividends. Ask a successful lawyer who's been divorced at least once about the cost of a divorce. (Or better yet, ask a family law attorney.) Sure, the divorce may have resulted from making a wrong choice of partner from the outset, but more often than not, it results from not allocating the time, energy, and resources required to cultivate a great marriage. Lawyers who practice law within a wellness lifestyle understand the foundational role that a love relationship plays in their quality of life, and they do the things required to solidify that foundation daily.

Or what about the lawyers who must spend tens of thousands of dollars on health procedures to treat a preventable chronic illness? Many lawyers, in the first two-thirds of their life, spend their health to gain their wealth, and in the last third of their life, spend their wealth to gain their health. Will you be one of them? Or will you invest in your health now so that you can reap the rewards of time freedom, financial freedom, *and* health freedom in your later years?

In this chapter, I highlighted the main benefits that a wellness lifestyle can deliver to lawyers, both in terms of their career and in their overall life. The rest of the book is about what you need to know and do in order to achieve those benefits. The next chapter looks at the concepts of health, happiness, and fulfillment, and at the reasons so many lawyers struggle to achieve these three things that are essential to a high quality of life.

2

THE 3 UNS: WHY MANY LAWYERS ARE UNHEALTHY, UNHAPPY, OR UNFULFILLED

Despite the powerful forces that seemingly collude and conspire against it, each of us is meant to live a healthy, happy, and fulfilling life. If you are a lawyer—and I assume you are if you are reading this book—then I want to be crystal clear from the outset that yes, I am talking about you, too. Not only *can* your life be full of health, happiness, and fulfillment while practicing law—it is *meant* to be.

Think about it for a moment. Why else would you be put on this Earth? Do you think that whoever is running the Universe—be it God, Nature, Source, or Whatever—has really set out to make us unhealthy, unhappy, and unfulfilled? Of course not. We were not put on this planet to experience sustained misery. We were put on it to express health, happiness, and fulfillment. We are here to fulfill our potential, to experience joy and love and passion, and to make the world a better place for those around us and for those who will follow after us.

That is not to say that every single moment of every single day is supposed to be bursting with joy and satisfaction. Life has its highs and lows—that is in part what makes it interesting and worth living. But chronic illness, sustained unhappiness, and ever-elusive fulfillment? No way. That isn't the master plan. If you think it is, then you probably need to read this book more than anyone.

So we have a problem. We are meant to be healthy and happy and fulfilled, but the evidence shows that many, many lawyers are not as healthy, or happy, or fulfilled as they would like to be. Worse, many lawyers experience two or all three Uns: They are unhealthy, unhappy, *and* unfulfilled. That is not a fun way to experience your short time on this planet.

This chapter will discuss the roles that health, happiness, and fulfillment (and the lack thereof) play in our lives. It will survey the data relating to the health, happiness, and fulfillment of lawyers, and it will examine some of the probable and possible causes of that data. Finally, it will propose a cure for the 3 Uns, which will lead in to the remainder of the book.

While this chapter examines each of health, happiness, and fulfillment separately, it's important to note that each is interconnected with the others. Generally, healthy people are happier; it's no fun to be sick. If you're unfulfilled, that's going to affect your happiness, too—it's difficult to be full of joy when you know in your gut that you're just not making the difference in the world that you want to be making, or if you're certain you're not reaching your potential. And happiness and fulfillment are key aspects of mental, emotional, and spiritual wellbeing, which we'll see are requirements to experience optimal health. So as we look at each of health, happiness, and fulfillment separately, keep in mind that the boundaries between them are fluid.

HEALTH

What is health?

The World Health Organization (WHO) defines health as follows: *Health is a state of complete physical, mental, and social well-being, and not merely the absence of disease or infirmity.*

The first thing that jumps out to many when they read this definition is that health is more than simply not being sick—the absence of disease or infirmity. That's part of it, but health goes beyond that. It involves complete wellbeing in three vital areas of life: physical, mental, and social. Essentially, in order to be healthy, you need to have a healthy body, a healthy mind, and a healthy relationship with the people and the world around you. That is no small matter.

Many people, lawyers included, mistakenly equate health not to an absence of disease or infirmity, but to an absence of symptoms. *No pain? I'm good. No aches? No problem.* However, if you're ache- and pain-free, but start to wheeze after walking up two flights of stairs, are you healthy? If you're ache- and pain-free, but you take a couple of prescription drugs every day, are you healthy? If you're ache- and pain-free, but you're stressed to the max day after day, are you healthy? We'll look at these questions in greater detail in the next chapter, but the short answer to each, according to the WHO definition of health, which requires *complete* physical, mental, and social well-being, is no.

Where does health come from?

The World Health Organization lists the following factors as the key determinants of health[10]:

> ➢ Income and social status
> ➢ Education
> ➢ Physical environment (i.e. safe water and clean air, healthy workplaces, safe houses, communities, and roads)
> ➢ Social support networks
> ➢ Culture
> ➢ Genetics
> ➢ Personal behavior and coping skills
> ➢ Access to health services
> ➢ Gender

It is interesting to note that with respect to healthy workplaces, the WHO states that people who have more control over their working conditions tend to be healthier than those with less control. Lacking control over their work requirements is a major issue experienced by lawyers, particularly junior lawyers. This not only can affect health, but happiness as well.

It is evident in looking at the WHO's list of the key determinants of health that health is indeed a holistic issue. There are physical, intellectual, and emotional aspects to it, and not all of it is predetermined by our genetics. In fact, as will be discussed in detail in the next chapter, for the vast majority of us, genetics has very little to do with our health outcomes. By far the biggest influencer of health outcomes is your lifestyle—or, in the words of the WHO, your behavior patterns and coping skills.

The WHO notes in relation to the determinants of health that the "context of people's lives determines their health, and so blaming individuals for having poor health or crediting them for good health is inappropriate. Individuals are unlikely to be able to directly control many of the determinants of health."[11]

I believe the WHO has it wrong here. While it may not be appropriate to blame, neither is it appropriate for people to relinquish responsibility over their health. In saying that people are unlikely to be able to control many of the determinants of health, the WHO is paying too little attention to what you *can* control, which is your pattern of behavior, your daily choices, and your actions—in essence, your lifestyle. Yes, you might not control the state of the economy, or the quality of your education as a youngster, but you can—and must—take responsibility over your level of health. (This applies to your happiness and fulfillment, too.) I will save a deeper exploration of this vital issue for the next chapter.

The health of lawyers

In his wonderful essay *On Being a Happy, Healthy, and Ethical Member of an Unhappy, Unhealthy, and Unethical Profession,* Patrick J. Schiltz writes that "the few researchers who have studied the legal profession are unanimous that lawyers are, as a group, in remarkably poor health."[12]

Are lawyers less healthy than the general population? It's tough to say. What we do know is that the general population isn't very healthy. If you live in the United States or Canada, you just have to spend ten minutes in the nearest public place to see evidence of our growing obesity epidemic. And if you're not aware of the soaring rates of heart disease, diabetes, cancer, and other chronic illnesses in most industrialized nations, then you really have been working too hard!

In this respect, it isn't terribly useful to determine if lawyers are healthier or less healthy than non-lawyers, since we all live in a society marked by a health crisis and we're all very much a part of it.

Most studies and surveys that have looked at the health of lawyers have focused on mental, and to a lesser extent, emotional health. For example, in an oft-referenced Johns Hopkins University study of more than 100 occupations, researchers found that lawyers have the highest incidence of depression in America. Lawyers also suffer exceptionally high rates of alcoholism and suicide.[13]

An article appearing on health.com rated a career in law as one of the worst jobs for your health, alongside transportation workers, enlisted soldiers, manual laborers, health care shift workers, and emergency services personnel.[14] The article cited stress and depression levels amongst lawyers as the reason for the poor ranking.

The focus on mental health issues is understandable given that the profession is known to create high levels of stress for its practitioners, and the fact that most people consider chronic stress to be a mental health issue only; they discount or fail to fully acknowledge the devastating physical effects caused by chronic stress.

Plus, collecting physical health data on a group as diverse as lawyers is difficult—it is impractical to get a wide cross-section of lawyers to participate in physical testing and third-party lifestyle assessments. So the information we have on the physical health of lawyers is mostly self-reported, i.e. not overly reliable. It's human nature to inflate how good things are and to minimize how bad things are when you're self-assessing. It's no fun to admit your shortcomings, even when surveys are anonymous.

For instance, in a 2012 Canadian Bar Association (CBA) survey of 1180 lawyers on wellness issues[15], almost 70% of respondents said they have excellent or good physical well-being and mental/emotional well-being. A full 67% said they always or often eat a healthy, balanced diet! Does that jive with your experience? As with most surveys, the question is everything. What constitutes a healthy, balanced diet? Making sure that 50% of every meal consists of locally grown, organic vegetables, and minimizing refined sugar? Eating fast food no more than three times a week? Following government-approved Food Guide recommendations to a T?

More importantly, what constitutes well-being? Is it a lack of symptoms? Is it complete physical, mental, and emotional well-being, to use the words of the WHO? Is it experiencing a high degree of health and vitality in all dimensions of life? Clearly, what constitutes well-being, and what a healthy diet consists of, can vary greatly from lawyer to lawyer, so the survey results must be digested accordingly.

That said, there are a great many lawyers who *do* experience high levels of physical, mental and emotional well-being. So there are role models in our profession who we can learn from and who prove that experiencing one or more of the 3 Uns is not a necessary component of the practice of law.

Yet, for all of the positive self-assessed statistics reported in the CBA survey, in its questions relating to other members of the profession, the picture isn't as rosy. When respondents were asked if they or a lawyer they know has experienced any of a series of wellness-related issues, the numbers were a little more dire:

➢ Stress/burnout issues – 92%
➢ Anxiety – 84%
➢ Depression – 76%
➢ Physical health issues – 74%[16]

These statistics point to the conclusion that the profession can and does lead to health issues for many lawyers—just not for most of the lawyers that complete the surveys, evidently.

Why many lawyers are unhealthy

Remember, the general population is in a health crisis, so any negative health trends among lawyers must be viewed in that context. When looking at negative health outcomes among lawyers, generally it's not an intelligence or socio-economic issue—although certainly there are uninformed and financially challenged lawyers amongst our ranks. The vast majority of us know that health is important in our lives, and in order to be healthy, we need to exercise regularly, consume a healthy diet, and manage our stress levels. We all have varying degrees of knowledge about *how* to do these things most effectively, but we know they're important and that they should be done.

So why do so many of us *not* do these things on a consistent basis? Well, it's mainly because it's hard to do them. It's easier to sit on a couch than it is to go for a 20-minute jog. It's easier to pick up fast-food at the drive thru on the way home than it is to plan, purchase, and prepare healthy meals and snacks. It's easier to let the demands of our career run rampant and trample other aspects of our lives (our happiness and fulfillment included) than it is to proactively instill boundaries on our career and to uphold them with conviction when most of our colleagues and clients test those boundaries every day. But as the great personal development gurus often say, life can be easy-hard, or hard-easy. In other words, life can be a little bit easy now and a lot harder later, or it can be a little bit hard now and a lot easier later. The decision is up to you.

Another reason that many lawyers are unhealthy is simply because they don't invest enough time and attention to their health; they don't value it highly enough. Many lawyers pay much more attention to their investment and retirement portfolios than they do to their health. The irony, of course, is that retirement funds don't do you much good if you're too ill or infirm to really enjoy them—or worse, if you're dead. As the old adage goes, if you don't make time for health now, you'll have to make time for illness later.

To be fair, moreso than most professionals, lawyers have less time and more stress to deal with. So it's even harder for lawyers to fit in the time for exercise, eating right, and stress management than it is for most other people. But I don't think any of us entered the practice of law because it was going to be easy, right? There's no hiding the fact that lawyering is a tough gig. Hours can be long. Issues can be difficult. Clients can be unreasonable. Deadlines can be short. But as demanding as the practice can be, it can be equally rewarding. Helping your clients achieve a desired result can be a gratifying process and often produces a sense of accomplishment and fulfillment. And there are many other great aspects to the practice of law as well: intellectual challenges, financial rewards, and the opportunity to make a positive impact in your community or, in some cases, on society as a whole. The list could go on. But if you, as many lawyers do, often put client demands and necessities ahead of your own, then invariably, over time, the result is not pretty. Health is compromised. Relationships end. Quality of life decreases. Stress rules the day. If you aren't healthy enough to enjoy the rewards of practicing law—financial and otherwise— then what's the point?

Another major irony when it comes to lawyers and health is that, particularly in the billable hour world, you tend to get paid in significant—if not direct—proportion to how *much* you work. And when you're not healthy, you can't work. Or, I should say, you shouldn't work—many lawyers do work through significant health issues even though they should be resting and recuperating. When this happens, everyone loses. The lawyer loses by not allowing him or herself to do what's necessary to get healthy. The lawyer's family loses because their loved one is inching closer to permanent disability or death. The client loses because, despite the fact that we like to think of ourselves as superheroes, it's impossible to remain focused and effective in the practice of law if you're battling physical, mental, or social health issues. The billable hour model masks this to a certain extent since it rewards inefficiency. But that is a short term, unsustainable view. Sooner or later clients will realize that the quality and value of your services just isn't good enough and they will move on to another lawyer for their legal needs. Plus, as discussed in the last chapter, the billable hour is in the twilight of its legal career anyway. In this respect, when a lawyer continues to practice when not healthy, he or she may continue to make money, but the profession ends up with another tick in the loss column.

One final factor that contributes to negative health outcomes among lawyers is that many lawyers aren't happy in their careers and in their lives. As the authors of a book on the subject of lawyer happiness have noted, "[h]appiness makes us healthier. It produces better immune systems and makes us more resilient when we suffer setbacks. Happy people live longer than unhealthy people."[17]

So let's move on to look at the concept of happiness and to consider the question *Are lawyers happy?*

HAPPINESS

What is happiness?

The dictionary definitions of happiness include feeling pleasure, contented, and satisfied. Happiness manifests itself in different forms; what makes one person happy can make another cringe. The recipe for experiencing happiness is different for all.

The pursuit of happiness is relatively new as a central goal of life. In modern times, when most of the population no longer has to worry on a daily basis about acquiring the basic necessities of survival, we have more time and inclination to pursue happiness. The flip side, of course, is that when our pursuit of happiness isn't going so well, we have more time and inclination to experience unhappiness.

Happiness has become a much researched and written about subject in recent years.[18] Concern about the happiness of lawyers is also new, arising as a result of surveys that show the declining happiness levels of members of our profession. That concern has given rise to some scholarly writing on the subject. Nancy Levit and Douglas O. Linder wrote an entire book about it called *The Happy Lawyer: Making a Good Life in the Law*. It offers a wealth of information on the art and science of happiness as it applies to lawyers.

Despite the relatively newfound role of happiness in modern society, some pretty smart people have talked about the importance of happiness for thousands of years. Aristotle, for instance, said that "happiness is the meaning and purpose of life; the whole aim and end of human existence." It doesn't get much more profound than that.

The Happy Lawyer authors point out that there are different kinds of happiness. There's short-term happiness akin to feeling pleasure in the moment; there's long-term happiness akin to feeling that your life has been well-lived; and there's an intermediate sort of happiness that relates mostly to a feeling of general contentment with your life. While each has its place, and the boundaries between each are hazy, when most people talk of happiness they're referring to this third, intermediate, contentment sort of happiness.

Where does happiness come from?

While genetics play a role in happiness levels, how happy we are to a large degree is under our control. Our happiness, like our health, is largely the result of our lifestyle—our choices and actions. *The Happy Lawyer* authors conclude that the biggest influencers on happiness are family relationships, employment status, health and quality of government.[19] Perhaps we cannot directly control the quality of our government, but we *can* control to a significant degree the quality of our health, our career, and our relationships. In other words, happiness can be thought of "as a skill, not fundamentally different than learning to play the violin or learning to play golf."[20]

While you probably know some lawyers who seem as if they aren't happy unless they're stressed out—you might even be surrounded by them—chronic stress is not only bad for your health, it's bad for your happiness, too. Stress releases the hormone cortisol, which is the perfect short-term response to a stressful stimulus. However, elevated levels of cortisol are not supposed to be a long-term thing, as is the case with lawyers under chronic stress. As Levit and Linder note, "[w]hen this hormone is coursing through the brain in significant quantities, we can't be happy."[21] Two proven ways to reduce stress and to increase happiness are exercise and meditation, each of which will be discussed later in the book.

Contrary to popular belief among lawyers, one thing that has very little causal relationship with happiness is money. In the words of one Harvard psychologist: "We think money will bring us lots of happiness for a long time, and it actually brings little happiness for a short time."[22] Fact is, the income of most lawyers exceeds $50,000 per year, the amount above which research has shown money matters little to happiness.[23]

So can we conclude that money doesn't buy happiness? My view is that money doesn't guarantee happiness, but money can be used to pay for things that can make you happy. Marketing guru Joe Polish has said that he wants to have lots of money for things that money *can* buy—it might not be able to buy health and happiness directly, but it can buy some things that can increase your health and happiness. It might not be able to buy you love, but it can be used to buy things that can enhance a love relationship. Really the question is, *what do you have to do to acquire the money?* If the price you have to pay to acquire money requires constant sacrifice to your health and happiness, no amount of money can replenish those things after the fact. The key is to be happy doing the things that produce money.

Jon Butcher, one of the world's great quality of life engineers, has a very unique and empowering formula for happiness. In his view, happiness lives in the balance between *striving for more* and *being grateful for what you have.* Butcher argues that mastering the relationship between these two things is the key to happiness. This is because when you're grateful for what you have already, your motivation to achieve more (whether it be more money, or more of anything else in life) isn't just about *having* more, it's also about the *process* of creating more. He writes: "If you're not enjoying the process while creating abundance in all the important areas of your life, you're missing the point!"[24] And the point, according to Butcher, is happiness.

Amiram Elwork, Ph.D., Director of the Law-Psychology Graduate Training Program at Widener University, would agree. He writes in his book *Stress Management for Lawyers* that, "the best synonym for 'success' is 'happiness.' No matter what you have achieved professionally or financially, you cannot call yourself successful unless you are happy."[25]

The happiness of lawyers

A recent study showed that being an associate attorney is the unhappiest job in America.[26] It doesn't get much more stark than that.

However, in *The Happy Lawyer*, the authors reviewed several studies relating to the happiness of lawyers and found that the answer to question, *Are lawyers happy?* is more complicated than yes or no. Some are happy, and some are not. Age, seniority, type of practice, income, gender, and other factors all play a role and have at least some predictive correlation to our happiness levels.[27]

Studies show that public sector lawyers tend to be happier than those in private practice, and of those in private practice, the larger the firm the less happy lawyers tend to be. Since big firm lawyers generally make more money than their smaller firm counterparts, this provides further evidence that more money does not necessarily correlate with more happiness. Indeed, for many lawyers working in big firms, the opposite appears to be true.

Lawyers who have been practicing for a decade or more tend to be happier than those with less experience. Female lawyers who have children tend to be unhappier than male lawyer parents and any lawyer without children. This is attributed to the fact that moms feel the brunt of work life and family life pressures more than dads.

So if you're a childless lawyer working in the public sector and have 10-plus years of experience, then you must be super-duper happy! And if you're a mother working as a junior associate in Big Law, you must be downright miserable!

Of course, it's not that simple. There are plenty of happy lawyers across the legal profession, but there are plenty of unhappy lawyers, too. If you're a lawyer who regularly experiences unhappiness in your life, let's look at some of the possible reasons why.

Why many lawyers are unhappy

One reason why many lawyers are unhappy is that—and this is my favorite quote from *The Happy Lawyer*—"Lawyers are merchants of misery."[28] Lawyering isn't happy work. Most of the time, clients come to us when they have problems to solve. Generally, people who have problems aren't very happy, so the clients we're dealing with often aren't all that happy. And the problems they need help with—the problems that we get paid to take on for them—aren't happy problems. In many instances, lawyers help clients deal with a loss—of health, of family, of money, of employment—and these aren't often jolly issues to be knee-deep in every day.

Another argument to explain the unhappiness of lawyers comes from the field of positive psychology. Martin Seligman, Ph. D., a leader in the field, believes that one of the main psychological explanations for lawyer unhappiness is the high value placed on *pessimism* in the profession. Seligman notes that this isn't "glass half empty" pessimism, but rather pessimism in the sense that a pessimist views bad events as pervasive, permanent, and uncontrollable. According to Seligman's research, pessimists do better at law, because "seeing troubles as pervasive and permanent is a component of what the law profession deems prudence. A prudent perspective enables a good lawyer to see every conceivable snare and catastrophe that might occur in any transaction."[29] While prudence and pessimism may make you a better lawyer, generally they don't make you a better person. As Seligman notes, "a trait that makes you good at your profession does not always make you a happy human being."[30]

The authors of *The Happy Lawyer* write that there are six experiences central to happiness in the life satisfaction sense: security, autonomy, authenticity, relatedness, competence, and self-esteem.[31] Two of these are big reasons for widespread unhappiness among junior lawyers: autonomy and competence. It has often been said that law school is not called lawyer school for a reason; it might teach you the law, but it doesn't teach you much about being a lawyer. The first few years in practice involve a near vertical learning curve, and virtually no control over the type of work you do or how long you're expected to take to do it. Most associate lawyers learn pretty quickly that, after cancelling weekend plans the first two or three times, it's best not to make weekend plans at all. That's not much of a happiness generator.

Throughout one's legal career, there is a constant chase to be just the right amount of busy. We are all versions of Goldilocks looking for the level of busy-ness that is just right: not too busy, but not idle, either. In reality, most lawyers spend most of their careers swaying on the pendulum from being too busy to being not busy enough. Each is stressful in its own way, and as mentioned above, it's difficult if not impossible to experience much happiness when under chronic stress.

Authenticity, which can be described as living life in accordance with your values, is another driver of happiness. According to *The Happy Lawyer*, "[w]hen your goals are consistent with your deepest values and not the values someone else chooses for you, your life has a clarity and sense of purpose that makes achieving happiness much more likely."[32] Most lawyers don't have any sense of what their deepest values are and thus don't have any way of knowing whether they're living in accordance with them—other than the one major symptom that points in that direction: unhappiness. In this respect they lack a certain level of consciousness about what really matters in their life. As Ayn Rand said, "happiness is that state of consciousness which proceeds from the achievement of one's values." In the chapters that follow, this book will explore this concept further and will provide some guidance to help lawyers figure out what their values are and to create a life plan that will ensure they live congruently with those values. This is a skill that, as it turns out, lawyers are well-positioned to implement, as we'll see in Chapter 5.

There are many other causes of lawyer unhappiness. The emergence of mobile technology means that many lawyers feel they are never off the clock, and can never fully disengage from work no matter the time of day. Growing incivility in practice can erode whatever feelings of happiness lawyers may experience on the job; being the subject of verbal abuse or manipulative practices by opposing counsel isn't much fun. And a lack of balance between lawyers' personal and professional lives is cited as a major reason for lawyer unhappiness. This problem, and the solution for it, will be presented in greater detail in the chapters that follow.

FULFILLMENT

What is fulfillment?

As complex as the concepts of health and happiness may be, fulfillment is probably the most difficult to put in a box and tie a ribbon around. Whereas health refers mostly to the physical/mental aspects of our lives, and happiness is mostly mental/emotional, fulfillment is primarily emotional/spiritual. It enters a different realm of our lives. It relates to the bigger questions of *Why am I here? Does what I'm doing matter? Am I reaching my potential? Am I achieving my purpose?*

The dictionary says that fulfillment means to achieve something, to satisfy something, to complete something, or to realize ambitions. This is a good start. But to me, the real meaning of fulfillment begins to emerge when you look to a thesaurus for its list of synonyms. Serenity, self-actualization, gratification, inner peace, and nirvana are all on that list. Who doesn't want a little more of those in their life?

For many, fulfillment is the oft-forgotten stepsister of health and happiness. This is likely due to the fact that fulfillment is more of a long-term undertaking. There are lots of things you can do to improve your health and happiness in the next ten minutes (eat some vegetables, do some pushups, laugh with friends, buy a new pair of shoes) but there aren't many ways you can inject more fulfillment into your life in such a short span of time. And as we have seen, lawyers often aren't the best long-term thinkers out there. While you can be healthy and happy in the moment or for a short period of time, unless you are fulfilled, the happiness—and perhaps your health, too—will begin to erode.

Lest you think that *Why am I here?* and *Am I reaching my potential?* are purely esoteric questions that don't have much relation to the day-to-day world of practicing law, you should know that a sense of fulfillment is a basic human need. It's not an optional ingredient of the life you were meant to have; it's an essential one.

You're probably familiar with 20th century humanistic psychologist Abraham Maslow's hierarchy of human needs. The hierarchy is based on the fact that all humans have essential needs that can only be satisfied if the needs below them are satisfied first. At the bottom you have physiological needs such as food, water, and shelter. Next you have safety needs, followed by the feelings of belonging, love, and self-esteem. Do you know what's at the top of the hierarchy? Self-actualization and fulfillment. Yes, fulfillment is not only an essential human need, it's at the pinnacle of the needs pyramid. That means it's the most difficult to achieve—and the most rewarding.

ABRAHAM MASLOW
HIERARCHY OF NEEDS

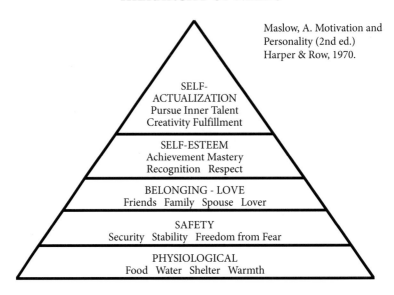

Maslow, A. Motivation and
Personality (2nd ed.)
Harper & Row, 1970.

SELF-
ACTUALIZATION
Pursue Inner Talent
Creativity Fulfillment

SELF-ESTEEM
Achievement Mastery
Recognition Respect

BELONGING - LOVE
Friends Family Spouse Lover

SAFETY
Security Stability Freedom from Fear

PHYSIOLOGICAL
Food Water Shelter Warmth

Maslow said that *"what human beings can be, they must be."* There is so much wisdom in that short, wonderful phrase as it relates to the human need for fulfillment and self-actualization. Philosopher and entrepreneur Brian Johnson writes of this phrase: "There is, in Maslow's language, a *need* you have to self-actualize—to live at your highest potential and to express your latent potentialities. If you don't fulfill this need, it's like depriving your soul of oxygen. Although you may not gasp as noticeably as you would if your more basic need of physical oxygen were deprived, you *will* experience equally (albeit more subtle) painful symptoms of angst, anxiety, depression."[33] Equating a lack of fulfillment with a lack of oxygen is a powerful image—one that brings the concept of fulfillment out of the long-term and into the present.

Where does fulfillment come from?

A sense of fulfillment comes from feeling that your work and your life matters, and that you are fulfilling your potential. It involves recognizing that you have been given a gift of life, and that you have an obligation to make the most of it. This may sound cliché, but then again this is a *need* we're talking about here. It's not an elective.

In *The Creative Lawyer: A Practical Guide to Authentic Professional Satisfaction*, Michael F. Melcher identifies the specific factors that make up a fulfilling career:

> ➤ The degree of match between your core values and what you do
> ➤ Vision and strategy
> ➤ Attention to relationships and consistent networking
> ➤ Mindful communications
> ➤ A habit of experimentation
> ➤ Parallel growth and lifelong learning
> ➤ A willingness to tolerate ambiguity
> ➤ Shaping your own story
> ➤ Openness to interrogating personal taboos[34]

Many of these factors are components of living a wellness lifestyle, and will be explored later in this book. The point of listing these factors here is not so that you memorize them and methodically implement them into your career forthwith, but rather to demonstrate that fulfillment—like health and happiness—isn't happenstance. There are things you can do and characteristics you can cultivate that can enhance the degree to which you experience fulfillment in your career and in the rest of your life.

The fulfillment of lawyers

If wanting or seriously considering a change in careers is evidence that many lawyers are not fulfilled, then there is no dearth of evidence to be found. Here's a sampler of statistics that point to a crisis of career fulfillment among lawyers:

> ➤ Seven in ten lawyers responding to a California Lawyers magazine poll said they would change careers if the opportunity arose.[35]
> ➤ One comprehensive longitudinal study found that just two years after graduation, almost 60% of big firm lawyers who

had graduated from top-ten law schools expected to leave the profession within the next two years.[36]

> Fewer than half of respondents to a 2007 survey of the American Bar Association said that they would recommend a career in law to a young person.[37]

> Only half of lawyers are very satisfied or satisfied with their work.[38]

Since one's career is such an important component of one's life, we can conclude that many of the lawyers who are dissatisfied with their careers in law are not fulfilled in life, either.

Why many lawyers are unfulfilled

As *Lawyer Bubble* author Steven Harper writes, "[f]or the profession and for society generally, it's important to understand why so many lawyers find themselves in unfulfilling careers."[39] A major reason why many lawyers are unfulfilled in their career is that they feel that their work doesn't matter. Matter, here, refers to mattering on a couple of levels. Often the legal work carried out by junior lawyers, especially at larger firms, doesn't have a clear connection to the bigger picture of the particular client file—at least none that is apparent to the junior lawyer. When you can't identify that the work you are doing is meaningful or has any significant value in moving the client's position forward, that tends to sap your level of fulfillment. This is especially true for lawyers who don't get much inherent value in writing memos on obscure areas of the law, preparing discovery or deposition summaries, or sorting through mountains of documents to identify whether they are privileged or not—especially if you're doing this kind of work at 3:00 a.m. As one lawyer aptly described, "a nice income doesn't deaden that kind of suck from one's life force."[40]

Mattering also means mattering in the context of contributing to the social good. Many new lawyers think their work in the law will make a difference in the world, but few new lawyers—few lawyers, period—feel that they actually do. One study found that only 16% of lawyers find that their career affords the ability to contribute to social good as much as they expected.[41] As Harper writes, in particular of big firm life, "the gap between a new law school graduate's expectations and the reality of life as a young associate is especially sizable."[42]

Feeling like you're working in a profession that, at best, isn't appreciated and, at worst, is viewed with derision by the public doesn't do much to fill up your fulfillment tank either. Lawyer jokes are funny—until they're not. We're pretty much the only profession with our own brand of jokes. Since they're all at our expense, it's not something to be particularly proud of. Neither is this: In a 2013 poll of 4,000 Americans, lawyers ranked last among 10 professions for contributions to society.[43] It is perhaps understandable that lawyers ranked a country mile behind members of the military and teachers in terms of contributions to society. But in an era marked by perceived corporate greed and questionable ethics among members of the mass media, that we ranked well behind journalists and business executives as well certainly isn't a feather in our collective cap.

Not finding over the moon fulfillment in your career doesn't necessarily mean that you lead an unfulfilling life. As will be discussed further in Chapter 7, your life's purpose doesn't have to coincide with your career's purpose. It's wonderful if it does, but it's not essential. One's fulfillment in life can come in a myriad of ways outside of law practice, whether that's to be a wonderful spouse, parent, community leader, or volunteer, or through the competition of sports, or the creativity of music or art. The list could go on and on. But the time pressures of practicing law often prevent lawyers from engaging in those other fulfilling experiences, activities, or pursuits. This generates more resentment in their career, which creates more stress—and often creates less time for these other interests. It's the proverbial vicious cycle and it is yet another reason why many lawyers are unfulfilled in law and in life.

WHAT'S THE SOLUTION?

So what can you do to enhance your degree of health, happiness, and fulfillment? How do you solve the Great Lawyer Riddle?

The answer isn't waiting for the profession to change. Change is coming, yes, but as discussed in Chapter 1, that change isn't going to make lawyering any less stressful. The three major drivers of change in the profession—the "more-for-less" challenge, liberalization, and exponentially evolving technology—all will make the practice *more* competitive and *more* stressful for most lawyers. The changes on the horizon will force lawyers to be much more innovative and effective, to embrace new business models and new ways of delivering legal services. The legal marketplace is going to get tougher, and those unprepared will continue to suffer one or more of the 3 Uns on a sustained basis.

As mentioned in the last chapter, it's not the profession's job to ensure that you are healthy and happy and fulfilled. Yes, it's likely that part of your national bar association's purpose is to foster a high quality of life for its members, but let me ask you this: How is it doing so far? It has been my experience that bar associations are generally unwilling to grant CLE accreditation to proactive wellness programs, unable to see how improved wellness helps lawyers achieve a higher quality of life—not to mention a higher degree of professionalism. Like most governing bodies, bar associations are mostly reactionary. They tackle issues after they have arisen. While most, if not all, bar associations have identified that many of their members have quality of life issues, the majority of them don't know how to deal with that effectively. Many have the usual exercise, eat right, and manage stress resources on their websites which, granted, is better than nothing. But in my experience, lawyers don't spend a whole lot of their time surfing bar association websites. Similarly, lawyer assistance programs are helpful, but they are typically "call us when you're in trouble" resources that don't do much to prevent issues from arising in the first place.

Neither is the solution to the Great Lawyer Riddle found by looking to your law firm or employer to enhance your health, happiness, and fulfillment. Yes, they certainly have a role to play, and any firm or employer with any degree of thinking beyond next week will offer wellness programs to their lawyers and staff. But few have figured out a way to actually get many of their lawyers to *use* the wellness programs or to participate in the wellness initiatives they have implemented.

The only solution to the Great Lawyer Riddle—the only path to enhanced, sustained health, happiness, and fulfillment—is for you to take on the responsibility yourself by fully adopting and implementing a *wellness lifestyle*. As we'll see in the next chapter, health, happiness, and fulfillment are the *effects* of living a wellness lifestyle. You cannot experience all three on a sustained basis without doing so. The good news is, as we'll see in Chapter 3, you can exercise a greater degree of control over your lifestyle— and therefore your health, happiness, and fulfillment—than you probably realize.

3

LIVING A WELLNESS LIFESTYLE

My father-in-law likes to tell a story about a lawyer lost for days in the desert. The lawyer is clinging to his life, half-delirious and stumbling, searching for water. At last he comes across a nomad whom he begs for water. "I don't have any water," says the nomad, "but I can give you a necktie." "A necktie," gasps the parched wanderer, "I don't need a necktie! I need some water!" And on he stumbles. As luck would have it, he comes across another nomad a short time later, and again he begs for water. "I haven't any water," says the second nomad, "but I have a necktie for you." "What is wrong with you people," exclaims the lost, dying lawyer, certain the next hour will be his last if he doesn't find any water to drink. A short time later, just before he is about to resign himself to his fate and pass out for good, he spots some sort of mirage in the distance. Unsure if he is hallucinating, he finds the resolve to carry on a few hundred yards further, in the direction of the mirage. As he gets closer, he can't believe his eyes as a beautiful, breath-taking oasis emerges from the haze and presents itself to him. With the last ounce of energy the lawyer can muster from his dehydrated body, he crawls to the entrance of the oasis and asks the guard for some water. "Sorry sir," answers the guard. "You need a necktie to get in here."

It's not the best joke in my father-in-law's voluminous repertoire, but as an analogy for the importance of wellness for lawyers, it's spot on. The water the doomed lawyer so desperately wanted equates to our work as lawyers: our clients, our files, our billings, and our livelihood. Much like water to a lost man in a desert, our career as a lawyer sustains us, helps to give us life. But lawyers often disregard the fact that there is one thing that we need above all else in order to be in a position to have a career in the first place: our health. And just as the dying man disregarded the possible use of the necktie because he was so focused on water, lawyers too often disregard the foundational importance of a wellness lifestyle (the means to achieve health—not to mention happiness and fulfillment) in their lives. There is no career when there is no health. There is no water if there is no necktie.

THE MOST IMPORTANT LAW IN THE UNIVERSE

The most important law in the universe, for lawyers and non-lawyers alike, is the Law of Cause and Effect. The Law of Cause and Effect states that nothing in this universe happens by chance; every effect has a cause. Lawyers, more than most people, should be familiar with this concept. Trial lawyers deal with causation issues all the time. But I suggest that most lawyers—and most non-lawyers, too—fail to grasp that this law determines the degree to which you experience health, happiness, and fulfillment in your life. They don't fully grasp that your current levels of health, happiness, and fulfillment are the *effect* of your past choices and actions. Put another way, all of the choices and actions you have made in the past have combined to *cause* your current degree of health, happiness, and fulfillment.

The wonderful thing about the Law of Cause and Effect is that you *control* the choices you make and the actions you take. You control the causes in your life, and therefore you *own* the effects of those causes—be they desirable or undesirable. When it comes to your degree of health, happiness, and fulfillment, there is no random chance. The degrees to which you experience these things, as well as the overall quality of your life, are your responsibility.

Granted, it's a big responsibility. But isn't it empowering to know that you're not just a bystander when it comes to your health, happiness, fulfillment, and quality of life? You're at the wheel. You can take credit for a high degree of health, happiness, and fulfillment, and you must take responsibility if you experience one or more of the 3 Uns on a sustained basis.

So how do you create sustained health, happiness, and fulfillment in your life? There's only one way. It's by living a wellness lifestyle.

WHAT IS A WELLNESS LIFESTYLE?

What is a wellness lifestyle? In order to answer that question, one must first get clear on what wellness means. This is no easy task. Wellness is one of the most over-used and misused terms in the English language. Today there are wellness dog foods, wellness Botox centers, wellness pharmacies, wellness everything. There's even a Paranormal and Wellness Society in my hometown. I guarantee that the vast majority of people and companies that incorporate wellness into their business name or otherwise promote wellness in connection with their products or services have no idea what it means.

We're lawyers, so we need to define what we're talking about. Since we invented the term *defined term*, let's agree on a good definition of wellness before we move on.

About a dozen years ago, wellness visionary Dr. Patrick Gentempo set out to create the world's leading wellness brand. He called it the Creating Wellness Alliance. Today, there are more than 350 Creating Wellness Centres internationally. When Dr. Gentempo and his team created the Creating Wellness Alliance, there was no dictionary definition for the term wellness. They needed to create one. This is what his team came up with:

Wellness is the degree to which an individual experiences health and vitality in any dimension of life.

There are now dictionary definitions for wellness, and other definitions abound online. But Dr. Gentempo's is the best one available. It's simple, but profound. Here are three key components of the definition:

1. It implies that health and wellness are not the same thing. Wellness subsumes the concept of health and includes the concept of *vitality*.

2. By including the concept of *degree*, the definition includes the premise that wellness exists on a continuum; that is, we all have some degree of wellness, and our degree of wellness can increase or decrease.

3. It notes that there are different *dimensions* of life. This infers that we can experience a high degree of wellness in one dimension and a low degree of wellness in another.

I'll explore all of the different dimensions of wellness in the next chapter. For now, I'll discuss the other two concepts listed above, namely, the concepts of vitality and degree.

Vitality: the secret sauce of life

In the last chapter, we looked at the WHO definition of health: *Health is a state of complete physical, mental and social well-being and not merely the absence of disease or infirmity.* This definition of health—the idea that it is more than just the absence of disease— approaches what many people think of when they hear the term *wellness*; that is, a more positive and holistic outcome of physical, mental, and social well-being.

Yet there are two major differences between the terms health and wellness. First, health contemplates "complete" well-being. Wellness, as discussed above, is not an all-or-nothing affair. There are different *degrees* of wellness. The same is often said of health, but given the WHO's definition, that is inaccurate.

The second major difference between health and wellness is that wellness includes the concept of *vitality*. Remember the definition from above: *Wellness is the degree to which an individual experiences health and vitality in any dimension of life.* When you hear people talk about health and wellness, as if the two words cannot exist on their own, they haven't really thought through what the two terms mean. Wellness subsumes the concept of health, so if you're talking about wellness, you don't need to separately refer to health.

But don't go emailing your law firm's Health and Wellness Committee or the head of your bar association's Health and Wellness Section to tell them they must change the name forthwith. There's no harm done in lumping the terms health and wellness together so that they roll off the tongue as easily and unconsciously as cease and desist. As a lawyer, you spend enough time wrestling with language every day; you don't need an exercise in linguistics when you're reading in your spare time. The point I want to stress about the difference between health and wellness is the concept of *vitality.*

The dictionary defines vitality as liveliness, meaning abundant physical and mental energy, usually combined with a wholehearted and joyous approach to situations and activities. Vitality's synonyms include energy, strength, life, vigor, get-up-and-go, and joie de vivre. These are all beautiful things and symbols of a life well lived. And while they come close to describing accurately what vitality is, they still fall short. Vitality also includes the concepts of passion, purpose and love, and anything else that makes life worth living. Vitality is the secret sauce; without it we're not *fully* alive. Even more than health, the degree to which we have vitality is the degree to which we will experience a high quality of life.

The previous chapter discussed in detail the concepts of health, happiness, and fulfillment, and how they're integral to one's overall quality of life. Since wellness is the degree to which you experience *health and vitality* in your life, vitality, then, represents happiness and fulfillment in the context of wellness. When you are happy and fulfilled most of the time, you experience vitality; when you are chronically unhappy and unfulfilled, you do not. Whereas health is in many (but not all) ways objectively quantifiable through diagnostic testing, happiness and fulfillment are not. Vitality, just like happiness and fulfillment, cannot be fully and accurately measured. Nevertheless, you know on a guttural level if you have a high degree of vitality—and even more so if you don't.

So how do you get more of this vitality stuff in your life? What's the secret to obtaining the secret sauce? Well, as you might expect, there's no easy or one-size-fits-all answer to that question. A lot of it has to do with getting conscious about what all of the important areas or dimensions of your life *are,* and then making sure your daily choices and actions improve your degree of health and vitality in each area. In other words, sustained vitality—just like sustained health—comes from living a holistic wellness *lifestyle.*

Your lifestyle determines your degree of wellness

Wellness exists on a continuum, meaning that we all have some *degree* of wellness in our lives. In other words, *illness* is another way of saying that you have a very low degree of wellness.

Wellness is not static; it's always changing. Every day, as a result of the choices you make and the actions you take, you move further towards wellness or further away from it. *Every day.* Of course, short of a car accident, heart attack, or some other major health event, you won't notice that you move towards wellness or illness every day. You probably won't notice it in a week, a month—maybe not even a year. But it's happening. And even if *you* don't notice it, others might.

Dr. Deepak Chopra describes the concept this way: "If you want to know your experiences in the past, examine your body now [...] and if you want to know what your body will look like in the future, examine your experiences now."[44]

What Dr. Chopra is saying here is that your level of wellness is *not* the result of random chance or luck. It is the result of the choices you have made in the past, plain and simple. It is the result of your lifestyle.

The dictionary definition of lifestyle is *manner of living.* So what living a wellness lifestyle really means is a *manner of living that enhances your degree of health and vitality in all dimensions of your life.* Every single day counts. As author Annie Dillard said, "How we spend our days is, of course, how we spend our lives." This applies quite literally to the degrees of health and vitality that we experience in our lives.

Here is just a tiny sampling of the choices you make every day that impact your degree of wellness:

> ➢ Whether to exercise
> ➢ Whether to dip further into your credit line
> ➢ What to eat for lunch
> ➢ Whether to meditate

> ➢ How often you tell your spouse and kids that you love them
> ➢ How to handle a stressful situation
> ➢ What time to go to bed
> ➢ How much water to drink
> ➢ How many hours you work
> ➢ How much time you spend at a computer or in front of a television
> ➢ What kind of social interactions to engage in

The list goes on and on. Every one of those choices will take you further towards wellness or further towards illness. And notice how these choices don't all relate simply to exercise and diet. Those are important aspects of wellness, to be sure, but they're not the whole story. We'll look at the various dimensions of life in the next chapter.

There are three more important things to note about the wellness continuum, and thus, about living a wellness lifestyle. First, more important than where you are now on the continuum—your current degree of health and vitality—is the direction in which you're headed. You can't do anything now to change your past choices and actions, but you can control your choices and actions from this point in your life forward. You, and only you, control the direction in which you're headed. Will your choices and actions today move you further towards wellness, or farther away from it?

Second, striving to experience higher degrees of health and vitality in your life is not about perfection. It's essential to recognize, understand, and come to terms with the fact that you won't always make great choices—no one on the planet does. We're all human. Part of the experience of living is to make poor choices, so that we can learn from them and so that we can know the difference between success and failure, joy and sadness, and wellness and illness. If you've never been unhappy, how would you know the value of happiness?

Third, it's also important to understand that the same choice can enhance your level of wellness in one dimension of life, while decreasing it in another. Spending the weekend fishing with the boys might be great for your social wellness, but it also might be bad for the health of your marriage if it occurs weekend after weekend. Spending eight hours a day training for the next ironman triathlon might be great for your physical wellness, but it might be terrible for your career if you no longer have time to competently handle your job responsibilities. Eating a gigantic ice cream cone might not be great for your waistline, but if you're doing it while spending some real quality time with your daughter, that might be just what the doctor ordered for your family life. Just as in the practice of law, wellness isn't all black and white. It's not all either/or. The key is to know how your daily choices and actions impact your *overall* level of wellness, because more than anything else, it is the sum of your choices that determines your level of wellness and the quality of your life.

But how can you know how a choice or action will impact your overall level of wellness if you don't have a good handle on what all of the different dimensions of your life are? Most people don't—lawyers included. That's why the first step in living a wellness lifestyle is to purposefully think through and clearly articulate what your values and vision are for each dimension of your life. *What does my ideal level of health and fitness look like? What does my ideal marriage look like? What does my ideal career look like?* The next step is to create an action plan to consistently make the choices and do the things that are required to function at a high level in every important area of your life. The third step is to then actually make those choices and do those things. That is living a wellness lifestyle. That is a manner of living that cannot help but to enhance the degree to which you experience health and vitality across all dimensions of your life.

While at first blush you might think this is too difficult or unachievable, if you commit to it and avail yourself of the information, strategies, and resources in this book, you'll find it not only achievable, but easier than you think. You'll find it fun and exciting as well. And, as you'll discover in Chapter 5, if you're a lawyer, you already have the essential skillset to help you achieve this more easily than most others. Given the seemingly incessant demands of practicing law, this probably sounds counter-intuitive to you, I know, but you'll see that this is precisely the case in the chapters that follow.

WELLNESS AND AGING

Reproduced below is the wellness continuum developed by the Creating Wellness Alliance:

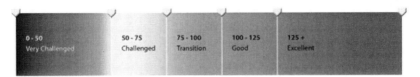

| 0 - 50 | 50 - 75 | 75 - 100 | 100 - 125 | 125 + |
| Very Challenged | Challenged | Transition | Good | Excellent |

This continuum uses a 200-point scale, with 100 being the score at which your chronological age (your age in years) and your biological age (the age of your body) are the same. Yes, chronological age and biological age are two very different things. The former is beyond your control, but you exhibit a great deal of control over the latter. We've all seen a 50-year old who looks 35, and a 50-year old who looks 65. Two 50-year olds, and one looks a full 30 years younger than the other. How does that happen? Is it because the younger-looking person has the "young-looking" gene and the older-looking person has the "old-looking" gene? Did the younger-looking person take the anti-aging pill that the older-looking person forgot? No, as we'll see below, neither genes nor drugs are the answer.

The answer is found in understanding that you are made up of a community of 50 trillion cells working together. Your cells are all identical, but they perform different functions. You have liver cells, and blood cells, and skin cells, and so on. Your individual cells are always reproducing; as "old" cells die off, new ones are produced to replace them. This is called cell division. You've probably heard that millions of your skin cells are shed and replaced every day, meaning that you develop a completely new layer of skin every month or two.

The important thing to know about cell division, at least with respect to its relationship to aging, is that there is a limit to how often your cells can divide in a lifetime. Experts have found that human beings can live for 120 years, meaning we are born with the capacity for our cells to keep dividing for that long.[45]

Yet we don't live that long. Our cells divide faster than that. The reason? *Stress.* Negative stressors in our lives cause cells to divide more rapidly. Examples of negative stressors include ingesting or inhaling toxic chemicals, eating a high sugar diet, feelings of anxiety, and so on. They also include the absence of what we need to express health: essential nutrients, regular exercise, feelings of love and belonging, and so on. So the more negative stressors that show up in your life, the faster you age. Who controls how many negative stressors show up in your life? You do. And the only way to minimize negative stressors in your life—the only way to exercise control over your aging process—is by living a wellness lifestyle.

Before we move on, take a moment to consider this: Where would you rate yourself on the wellness continuum?

Where would you like to be?

For many lawyers, answering the questions above can be difficult. It requires a reckoning of sorts. *Am I older than I should be? Am I aging too quickly? Can I really slow down the aging process?*

Yes, you can. Ask the 50-year old who looks 35—he did it.

WHAT ABOUT GENETICS?

Yeah, you might say (as many do), *but what about my genes? Will my daily choices and actions really make a difference if heredity isn't on my side?*

The misguided view that genes control health outcomes is probably the single biggest reason why so few people fully take responsibility over their level of wellness; why so few people fully adopt a wellness lifestyle. So often people say that they're bound to get this or that illness because one of their parents or someone in their family had it. You know the old story: *My dad had heart disease and died of a heart attack at 48, so I'll probably end up the same way.* If you think like that, you're not likely to adopt a wellness lifestyle, because, well, what's the point? If you think your health outcomes were predetermined the moment you were conceived, you won't be very inclined to adopt a lifestyle of daily choices and actions that enhance your degree of health and vitality. It would be like continuing to argue the case after the highest court in the land had handed down its ruling.

But your health outcomes *are not* predetermined. Genes *do not* control health. The *expression* of your genes does.[46] In the vast majority of cases, it's the environment in which the genes express themselves that is the key—not the genes themselves. As Ph.D. cell biologist and author Dr. Bruce Lipton describes it, "Genes are simply the molecular blueprints used in the construction of cells, tissues, and organs. The environment serves as a 'contractor' who reads and engages those blueprints and is ultimately responsible for the character of a cell's life."[47] In other words, your genes are the blueprint for your human house, but the quality of the blueprint matters little if the house is built by a poor contractor using subpar materials (bad food, no exercise, chronic mental or emotional stress, etc.). It's what you *do* with the genes you're born with that determines your degree of health and vitality. You control the expression of your genes; your genes don't control you.

Yes, there are some genetic diseases and illnesses. Down Syndrome is one example. If you have a 21st chromosome, you're going to have Down Syndrome 100% of the time. But that is the exception, not the rule, when looking at genes' predeterminative role in health outcomes.

Consider this: One hundred years ago, the most prevalent of the chronic illnesses that plague us today—heart disease, diabetes, obesity, cancer—barely even existed. Did the genetic code of human beings change during that time? Of course not. So it can't be genetics that causes chronic illness. It must be our lifestyle. In the words of renowned doctor of chiropractic and author Dr. James Chestnut: "If you actually study, and I have, and written about extensively, that if you actually trace the lifestyle changes of the human species over the last 100 years they completely explain entirely all the increases in chronic illness. If you trace the genetic changes over the last 100 years? They have no explanatory value at all. Zero."[48]

So if your dad died of a heart attack at 48, you might well end up the same way—but it won't be because of your genes. It will be because you adopted a similar lifestyle to your dad. It won't be your genes that kill you; it will be your lifestyle. As Dr. Chestnut notes, the number one killer of men and women today is not cancer or heart disease; it is suicide by lifestyle.[49]

But, you might say, my medical doctor told me I have a genetic predisposition for heart disease or some other chronic illness. That may be true. The genetic intelligence stored in your DNA may show something that makes you more likely to develop heart disease than the next person. But that doesn't mean you are going to develop heart disease. If you live an unhealthy lifestyle, that will trigger an unhealthy expression of your genes that will probably manifest as heart disease if you are predisposed to it. But if you live a wellness lifestyle and you give your cells a healthy environment in which to operate, your genes will express themselves accordingly and the predisposition won't manifest. You control the expression of your genes with your lifestyle.

Need more proof? Famed cardiologist Dr. Dean Ornish actually reversed atherosclerosis in a group of patients who adopted a regimen of exercise, healthy diet, and meditation.[50] The regimen didn't just slow down the development of the disease in these people—it reversed it. Why? Because living a healthier lifestyle caused the genes of the people in the study to express themselves in a healthier manner. In another study, Dr. Ornish showed that certain wellness lifestyle practices could alter the expression of over 400 genes in men with prostate cancer. Another study achieved similar results in women with breast cancer.[51]

It's the environment, stupid

Among other notable accomplishments, Dr. Bruce Lipton is a pioneer in the field of epigenetics, which has proven that when it comes to health outcomes, environment is the key, not genes. In his wonderful book, The Biology of Belief, Dr. Lipton cleverly entitled a key chapter It's the Environment, Stupid, as a play on President Clinton's economy-centered election campaign of the 1990s. By environment, Dr. Lipton doesn't mean the macro environment of the planet, although that can play a part. On a micro level—meaning your individual health—he's referring to the environment in which your 50 trillion cells reside. Are they given the essential materials they need to function properly, or are they operating in a deficient or toxic environment? Genes express themselves in accordance with the stimuli they encounter in their environment. Give the genes positive, health-enhancing stimuli like proper nutrition, regular exercise, and feelings of love and self-esteem, and your genes will express themselves in accordance with those positive stimuli. The reverse, of course, is also true. Give the genes negative, health-eroding stimuli like a poor diet, lack of exercise, and feelings of anxiety and stress, and your genes will express themselves in accordance with those negative stimuli. That negative stimuli—those negative stressors—will not only cause negative health outcomes, but they also, as discussed above, will increase your rate of cell division and will cause you to age more quickly.

Dr. Chestnut illustrates the environment versus genetics concept this way: If you see a pile of dead fish washed up on the shoreline, would you ask *what's wrong with their genes?* Or would you ask *what's in that water?* So why would it be any different with people?[52]

Yet in today's dominant healthcare paradigm, it *is* different with people. This bears further discussion.

PARADIGMS OF HEALTH

As mentioned above, scientific evidence demonstrates that the vast majority of chronic illness and disease today is caused by lifestyle factors and is preventable. In other words, we know that people who live a wellness lifestyle that includes healthy food choices, regular exercise, and management of mental and emotional stress are much more likely to express health and much less likely to express illness. We know that in the vast majority of cases, genes don't determine health outcomes—our lifestyle choices do. Only 5% of cancer and cardiovascular patients can attribute their disease to heredity.[53] Dr. Chestnut puts it this way: "We have this genetic blueprint, which we know is a sound blueprint. There's no evidence anywhere that maybe more than a maximum of two percent of people actually have genes that don't allow them to express health. Less than two percent according to the literature."[54]

So why, when someone gets sick or chronically ill, does our dominant health care model mostly ignore the importance of lifestyle in influencing health outcomes? When a patient presents with symptoms of illness or disease, rarely is an assessment of the patient's eating, exercise, and stress levels undertaken. Rather, more attention is paid to family histories and genetics. The medical doctor's objective is to diagnose what is "wrong" with the patient. When a patient presents with a symptom that deviates from the established norm of what constitutes being healthy (a blood pressure reading that exceeds the established healthy range, for example), the prevailing medical protocol isn't to try to assess what caused the high blood pressure or to consider what kind of lifestyle factors may be involved, but rather to take away the symptom. It's a pathological approach based on the idea that your body is not working properly because of faulty genes or because your body does not have the innate capacity to self-regulate and self-heal. This is the "allopathic" or "sickness and treatment" paradigm of health.

The sickness and treatment paradigm

As Dr. Lipton notes, the allopathic or sickness and treatment paradigm is centered on the theory that genes control health outcomes. This theory is called the *Central Dogma* by those who study and apply it. The problem with it is that it has never been proven. Dr. Lipton writes that "the notion that genes control biology has been so frequently repeated for such a long period of time that scientists have forgotten that it is a hypothesis, not a truth" and that "it has been undermined by the latest scientific research."[55]

A health care practitioner in the allopathic paradigm attempts to correct what is "wrong" with the patient with some sort of intervention, usually in the form of medication or surgery. In the case of cancer, this would include radiation and chemotherapy. If those interventions lessen or remove the symptoms of the patient, then that constitutes a successful outcome under this paradigm.

Since most medical doctors are trained under this allopathic paradigm, they are trained to diagnose and prescribe treatment for illness and disease; they are not trained to promote health or to prevent sickness. They are not trained in nutrition, exercise physiology, or stress management. They know that exercise, diet, and stress reduction are good for you, but because the foundation of their model is that genetics control health outcomes, they largely discount the role lifestyle plays not only in preventing illness and disease, but in treating them as well.

If genes did control health and there was nothing we could do to alter our health outcomes through our lifestyle choices, then using drugs and surgery to remove symptoms makes perfect sense. The allopathic paradigm is perfectly logical if you believe that illness is caused by bad genes or the body's inability to self-regulate and self-heal. If you can't do anything to change your health outcomes, then it makes sense to use interventions like drugs or surgery to make you more comfortable while living with the illness for the rest of your life. The toxicity of the drugs and/ or the invasiveness of the surgeries become necessary evils in the pursuit of the best quality of life possible, given the irreversibility of your genetically determined chronic illness.

The allopathic or sickness and treatment paradigm of healthcare can be summarized as follows:

> *Pathology*: Symptoms are a sign that the body is not working properly and that the body is not capable of self-regulation.
> *Genetics*: Genes control health outcomes. When a body is not working properly, it is a result of faulty genes or the body's inability to self-regulate.
> *Success = removal of symptoms*: Since we can't control our genes, and since the body can't self-regulate, the best course of action is to eliminate or reduce the symptoms through drugs, surgery, or other intervention.

It's an interesting paradigm. Even though we know that 98% of people are genetically able to express health if they create the right environment for their cells through healthy lifestyle choices, our dominant healthcare model treats everyone as though they're in the 2%!

Don't get me wrong; there is a fundamental need in our society for the diagnosing and treating of illness and disease. People are going to get sick, and we need highly trained, effective, and compassionate medical doctors to care for those people. We need that sick care system. Modern medicine is absolutely fantastic for crisis care and emergency care. If I am in a car accident tomorrow and suffer serious injuries and my life is threatened, I want an ambulance and I want medical doctors and surgeons to help piece me back together. Similarly, if I tear up my knee-playing hockey, I'm not going to go see my massage therapist or naturopathic doctor to fix my knee. I'm going to get an orthopedic surgeon to repair it. And if the pain after the surgery is unbearable, I'm going to take a painkiller to make me more comfortable for the short term. Let me be crystal clear: I am grateful for modern medicine and for the medical profession. I don't want to live in a society where I don't have access to those services when my loved ones or I require them.

But what about healthcare? What about removing the *cause* of symptoms rather than just the symptoms themselves? What about helping people to get well—to express a high degree of health and vitality—and not just symptom-free? Why do we not use the same methods to treat illness that we know are the keys to preventing it?

The wellness and prevention paradigm

There's another paradigm of health to consider. It's called the "wellness and prevention" paradigm. Its basic tenets are as follows:

- ➢ *Adaptive physiology*: Symptoms are a sign that the body *is* working properly; it is your body's inner wisdom, or innate intelligence, adapting to toxicities or deficiencies in its cellular environment.
- ➢ *Epigenetics*: Cellular environment controls the expression of your genes, and the expression of your genes controls health outcomes.
- ➢ *Success = removing the cause*: Since to a large degree we can control our cellular environment, and thus the expression of our genes, the best course of action is to eliminate the cause of symptoms through lifestyle change.

The fundamental principle of the wellness and prevention paradigm is that the body has an innate intelligence and that everything the body does, it does for a reason. If you don't believe that the body has an innate intelligence, think for a minute how you came to be; that is, from sperm and egg to human being. Think of what massive amount of intelligence was required to grow you from a single cell into a 50 trillion-celled organism in 40 weeks. Those of you who are parents like me have witnessed the miracle of childbirth. That miracle is innate intelligence at work.

If you subscribe to the wellness and prevention paradigm, when you get a symptom, you view it as your body telling you that it is under some stress—physical, biochemical, or psychological (more on the different kinds of stress in the next chapter)—that is foreign to the optimal function of the body. The symptom is a signal that you should identify those stressors and see if you can do something to eliminate them. The stressors cause the symptom. If you eliminate the stressors, you eliminate the cause, and you eliminate the symptom. Most times, you can do things to eliminate the stressors, such as getting lots of rest, increasing your intake of required nutrients, resolving an emotional problem in your life, etc.

To illustrate the point, I'll use a simple example. When your body gets a fever, what do you do? Do you view the fever as a bad thing; as something that must be treated with medication because there is something wrong with your body's ability to self-regulate? Or do you view the fever as a sign that your body is intelligently adapting to a stressor (a virus, for instance) in its cellular environment, by raising its temperature to combat that stressor? If the latter case holds true for you, instead of taking medication at the first sign of an elevated body temperature, you would probably get plenty of rest, increase essential nutrient intake, stay hydrated, monitor your temperature, and let your body's self-healing abilities go to work.

If you're not sure what to think about all of this, ask yourself this question: Is a fever caused by a lack of medication in your body?

When you apply this simple fever example to our society's chronic illness epidemic, you can begin to see how different the two paradigms are, and how the prevalence of one paradigm over the other has a profound impact on society. In the case of hypertension (high blood pressure), for example, if you decide to take medication to reduce the high blood pressure, then you're going to go down one path. You're going to try to trick your innate intelligence into thinking there's no problem. But here's the thing: Your innate intelligence can't be tricked—especially not for any length of time, like, say, years of renewed drug prescriptions.

But if you look at the high blood pressure as an expression of your body's innate intelligence and as a signal of an underlying cause or stress that needs to be dealt with, then you might look at your diet or exercise habits, or your level of emotional stress, and you might take some steps to change your lifestyle to eliminate the cause of the high blood pressure. That is quite a different path and, as Dr. Lipton, Dr. Chestnut, and other leading doctors and scientists have shown, it is a much healthier and much more empowering—not to mention scientifically validated—path to follow. Instead of taking blood pressure medication for the rest of your life, you might change your lifestyle and lower your blood pressure permanently, getting rid of the need for the medication altogether.

Can you imagine the impact on our society if everyone with chronic illness subscribed to the wellness and prevention paradigm of health, identified their symptoms as a call to action, and changed their lifestyle accordingly to eliminate the cause of those symptoms?

Better yet—can you imagine the impact on society if everyone adopted a healthy lifestyle from the outset, giving their body all of the nutrients and exercise it needed and avoiding toxic foods, chemicals, and lifestyle choices from Day 1 to prevent the vast majority of illness and disease in the first place? That is the world in which I want to live—and the world in which I want my children to grow up. That is one of the primary reasons I stopped practicing law and devoted myself full-time to helping lawyers achieve more health, happiness, and fulfillment. Because if lawyers—people who are known to have higher stress and less free time than most people—can do this; if lawyers can take the lead and become a profession of people committed to wellness and to improving their degrees of health and vitality, it would be the model for the world to follow. Let's create that world.

4

STRESS AND THE DIMENSIONS OF LIFE

In the last chapter, I looked at the definition of wellness and discussed that there are different dimensions of life. You can have a high level of wellness in one dimension of life while having a low level of wellness in another. If there were only one dimension of life, it would probably be pretty easy to live a wellness lifestyle. If, for example, career were the only dimension of life we needed to pay attention to, lawyers would probably lead the league in wellness!

I'm joking, of course, but the practice of law does have a way of taking over the rest of our lives unless we consciously take steps to stop that from happening. How easy it would be if there wasn't a "rest of our lives" to worry about, eh? But how sad would that be, too?

Thankfully, we don't have to imagine a world where a career is the only important aspect of life to concern ourselves with. There are many others that make up this thing called life. This chapter will discuss these different dimensions of life: All the stuff that can make life so hard, at times, but all the stuff that makes life worth living, too.

So what are these different dimensions of life? On the surface, it might not seem like one of life's big questions, but let me assure you that this is one of the most important questions you can ever ask. Getting a solid grasp on the different dimensions of your life, and how they impact your degree of wellness and the quantity and quality of your life, will do more to create health, happiness, and fulfillment than pretty much anything else you will ever do.

There are two ways to categorize the different dimensions of life. Both are important and instructive. The first is what I call the *physiological* dimensions of life, and the second is what I call the *social* dimensions of life.

THE PHYSIOLOGICAL DIMENSIONS OF LIFE

There are three physiological dimensions of life:

> ➤ *Physical*: How we move (or don't move) our bodies, i.e. exercise or lack thereof
> ➤ *Biochemical*: what we put in (or don't put in) our bodies, i.e. food, drink, drugs, etc.
> ➤ *Psychological*: how we think (or don't think), i.e. our beliefs, attitudes, self-esteem, etc.

These dimensions of life relate the types of *stress* that we experience in our daily lives. In other words, all of the stress you experience in your life falls under one or more of these three categories: physical, biochemical, and psychological.

Many lawyers are surprised to learn that stress isn't always a bad thing. Both positive and negative stress exists. Positive stress is also known as eustress, and negative stress is also known as distress. The chart below gives some examples of positive and negative stressors in each of the physiological dimensions of life.

Physiological Dimension of Life	Positive Stress (Eustress)	Negative Stress (Distress)
PHYSICAL	• Exercise • Good posture • Touch (massage therapy, chiropractic adjustment, etc.)	• Accident resulting in injury • Poor posture • Sedentary living
BIOCHEMICAL	• Intake of essential nutrients • Proper hydration	• Intake of toxic chemicals (in food, beverages, drugs, cigarettes, air, etc.)
PSYCHOLOGICAL	• Pressure to accomplish achievable commitment • Feelings of confidence, love, self-esteem, etc.	• Pressure to accomplish unachievable commitment • Feelings of being overwhelmed, loss of control, alienation, etc.

The most important thing you can know about stress is that all illnesses and injuries result from an excess of negative stress in one or more of the three physiological dimensions of life. Let me explain.

GAP and the stress response: Why we get sick

Each of us has something that Patrick Gentempo, D.C. calls General Adaptive Potential, or GAP for short.[56] Your GAP is your ability to process and dissipate stress in your daily life. When the level of negative stress in your life exceeds your body's ability to adapt to it, illness or injury results. Some people have a wider (higher) GAP and some have a narrower (lower) GAP, meaning that some have a higher ability to process and dissipate stress—and thus avoid illness and injury—than others. No, your GAP is not genetically predetermined; you have significant control over it, since it is an effect of how your genes are expressed and you control the expression of your genes with your lifestyle choices and actions. Being fit (physical), eating right (biochemical), and thinking well (psychological) will consistently increase your GAP; not doing those things will decrease it.[57]

While you can exercise control over your GAP, the width of your GAP has its limits. No matter how wide your GAP, there are some negative stressors that you won't be able to process and dissipate. For example, while urban myths may contend otherwise, you won't be able to survive a fall from 30,000 feet without a parachute. On the flip side, no matter how narrow your GAP, a paper cut probably won't kill you. But the vast majority of negative stressors that we experience in life fall on the spectrum between paper cut and free fall from an airplane, and your GAP will determine the impact those stressors have on your health. At your workplace right now, one of your colleagues probably has a cold or is carrying some other virus. Another of your colleagues will come into contact with that virus and will develop a cold. A third colleague will come into contact with that virus but will not develop a cold. The reason? The colleague who didn't catch the cold had a wider GAP than the person who did.

It's funny—when most people think of wellness, they tend to focus on exercise and eating right, and leave out attention to psychological stress. And when most people think of stress, they tend to focus on psychological stress, and leave out attention to physical and biochemical stress. But it's important to remember that all three physiological dimensions of life (and all three kinds of stress)—physical, biochemical, and psychological—greatly influence your quality and quantity of life. Decrease negative physical, biochemical, and psychological stress in your life, and you will proportionately enhance your level of wellness and, accordingly, your quality of life.

We get sick when the negative stress that we experience exceeds our body's ability to adapt to it. We'll all have some negative stress at any given point in our lives, but when negative stress accumulates it wears down our body's defenses, causing us to fatigue, get sick, and, eventually, die. Our body is great at adapting to stress (it's our innate intelligence at work), but the problem is that our body's stress response is only supposed to be a short-term adaptation. In other words, in the classic "fight or flight" example, our body adapts to the stress of being chased by a tiger by suppressing all systems in the body that are not essential in that moment for you to outrun that tiger (for example, your immune system, digestion, etc.). The body instead gives extra juice to all of the systems you need to outrun that tiger (for example, your respiratory system, cardiovascular function, etc.).

The key takeaway here is that the stress response is supposed to be short term. But so many lawyers today are under chronic negative stress—be it physical, biochemical, or psychological—because we don't treat our bodies and our minds properly. The result is that our bodies are in constant adaptation mode. Our immune system is chronically suppressed, our blood pressure may become chronically elevated, and so on. The body's adaptive capacity can handle this for so long—but only for so long—depending on your GAP. And your GAP, of course, is determined by your lifestyle.

Put another way, you don't get sick because of an absence of pharmaceuticals in your body. You get sick because, as Dr. Chestnut has written about extensively, there is toxicity and/or deficiency in your body.[58] You get sick because there are too many toxic elements in your life, like a poor diet, poor relationships, or high psychological stress, or because you are deficient in what your body needs to express health and vitality, like a nutrient-dense diet, regular exercise, or good self-esteem. You get sick because you have more toxic negative stress and/or insufficient positive stress than your body can process and adapt to at that time.

So the formula to prevent illness and to enhance your degree of health and vitality in life is pretty simple:

Minimize negative physical, biochemical, and psychological stress (toxicity and deficiency)

+

Maximize positive physical, biochemical, and psychological stress (purity and sufficiency)

=

High degree of wellness (health and vitality)

By now you know that the only way to achieve this is to live a wellness lifestyle. But that will include more than just paying attention to the three physiological dimensions of life. It is also essential to consider the social dimensions of life.

THE SOCIAL DIMENSIONS OF LIFE

The other way to look at the dimensions of life is to look at your life in the context of society. What are the different aspects or categories of your life that affect your ability to function in society at your highest level and to live your best life?

While the physiological dimensions of life are the same for everyone, the social dimensions of life may vary from person to person. Health will (or should) be on everyone's list of social dimensions. Family, career, and finances will apply to most people as well. Other social dimensions of life that merit some attention would be spirituality, intellect, mindset, emotions, community, and philanthropy. You can probably think of others.

Here's the thing: Most people don't know what the important social dimensions of their life are. They have never given much thought to it. This is tragic. Knowing what the social dimensions of your life are is the essential first step to functioning in society at your highest level, to living your very best life. Getting conscious of your social dimensions is a prerequisite for a life filled with health, happiness, and fulfillment.

Rethinking work-life balance

When I speak to law firms, bar association gatherings, or other lawyer groups, I often do an exercise that goes like this. I ask them who in the room actively pursues work-life balance, and who in the room believes that the practice of law involves too many demands for work-life balance to be a realistic goal to pursue. Most lawyers usually say they actively pursue work-life balance— probably because that's what they're told to do by the HR people and bar associations—while some of the more candid lawyers admit that work-life balance is not a realistic goal to pursue.

I then do something that no book on public speaking would ever recommend that speakers do: I tell them that they're *all* wrong. I tell them that the entire concept of work-life balance is based on the faulty premise that work and life are two separate things—that they exist apart from each other and can somehow achieve some sort of balance with each other. Of course, when you think about it, work and life cannot balance. Work is part of your life. You cannot balance a part with the whole. So while work-life balance is something we are encouraged to strive for in our lives at every turn, the concept doesn't make sense.

Then I acknowledge that the proponents of work-life balance really mean that you should try to achieve some sort of balance between your work and everything else in your life. I say that this makes a little more sense, and lawyers usually agree. Then I ask the lawyers to help me figure out what everything else in life actually is. I write "work/career" on the left side of a whiteboard, "everything else in life" on the right side, I put a line down the middle, and then I ask them this question: Other than work, what in your life is worth spending some time, energy, and resources on?

The first answer, almost always, is health. Other answers come quickly and plentifully, usually beginning with an "F." Family, friends, finances, faith, and fun. I write these on the right side of the whiteboard. Other responses from lawyers often include love, learning, relaxing, and hobbies—even pets. This is not an exhaustive list.

At the end of the exercise, the whiteboard looks something like this:

Work/Career	Everything Else in Life:
	Health
	Family
	Friends
	Finances
	Faith
	Fun
	Love
	Learning
	Relaxing
	Hobbies
	Pets
	Etc.

I then ask them this: Are you sure the goal we should be striving for is to balance work with *all* of this other stuff in our life? Does work *really* take up 50% of life's pie, with everything else lumped into the other half?

For many lawyers who do this little exercise, which takes all of about three minutes, it is the first time that they have ever really considered that your career is only one out of a number of important dimensions in your life. Very important, yes—but success there at the expense of other dimensions does nothing to improve your overall wellness or quality of life. Having a thriving law practice is great—but not at the expense of your health and fitness. Being healthy and fit is great—but not if your love relationship is all messed up. Being the world's greatest spouse is wonderful—but not if your financial life is a disaster. Sustained health and vitality requires success in every important aspect of your life. You need to operate at a high level in each of the social dimensions of your life. When you realize that, the faulty premise of work-life balance really comes into focus.

It's about LIFE balance

Of course, in order to achieve success across the spectrum of the social dimensions of your life, you will need to achieve some semblance of balance among all of those dimensions. By balance I mean devoting the time, energy, and resources to each dimension required to achieve success in that dimension. By balance I *do not* mean spending equal amounts of time, energy, and resources in each dimension—that would be not only impossible, but unnecessary. Some dimensions of your life—your career, especially, since you're a lawyer—are probably going to take more of your time than others. But—and this is the key—that doesn't necessarily make them more important than the other dimensions of your life. Renowned chiropractor and entrepreneur Dr. David Jackson coined the term "12 category smart" to describe the need to bring the requisite level of intelligence to the table in each of the 12 important social dimensions he identified in his life. Doing well in 11 categories just doesn't cut it; it only takes failure in one category to sink the whole ship. In much the same manner that oil spilling out of your neighbor's leaky oil tank won't stop seeping through the ground when it hits your property line, failure in *any* social dimension of your life will seep into all other dimensions of your life and contaminate them all. Problems in your love relationship will show up everywhere in your life. Problems with your finances will show up everywhere in your life. Problems in your career will show up everywhere in your life. And, of course, problems with your health will, too.

There are some who don't care for the term balance, either because it's too static to account for life's constantly changing circumstances, or for a myriad of other reasons. If you need to use some other word to own the concept being described here, that's okay. Some people like harmony, or flow, or whatever. Regardless of the word you want to use, the idea that you must operate at a high level in every dimension of life must be implicit in it. Achieving balance, harmony, or flow at a mediocre level just won't do it. You're meant to achieve health and vitality in every dimension of life, and that requires success across the board.

In an insightful article about quality of life issues faced by lawyers in the United States, former Minnesota law firm partner Patrick Schiltz presents an interesting take on the concept of life balance for lawyers. He argues that achieving some semblance of life balance is a requirement of practicing law *ethically*. In addition to complying with the formal rules of conduct applicable to lawyers as well as the informal rules of right and wrong governed by moral intuition, Schiltz says that to be an ethical lawyer you must live an ethical life. He writes that "being admitted to the bar does not absolve you of your responsibilities outside of work—to your family, to your friends, to your community, and, if you're a person of faith, to your God. To practice law ethically, you must meet these responsibilities, which means that you must live a balanced life."[59]

Schiltz goes on in the article to confess his personal failure to do so. "I had every intention of leading a balanced life," he writes, "and, by New York or Washington standards, I suppose I did. By anyone else's standards, I did not." He then recounts some life events he missed out on by travelling so much for work, such as his children learning to walk and talk, his grandmother's death, the time when the rest of his family was trapped by a winter storm, and the moment his wife found out that their unborn child had Down Syndrome. Looking back on his career in private practice, he concludes: "I failed miserably in my resolve to lead a balanced life, and neither my family nor I will ever be able to get back what we lost as a result."[60]

My "corporate" wellness chart

As mentioned, while the physiological dimensions of life are the same for everyone, the social dimensions of life may vary from person to person. We're all different, so we'll all have different areas of our life that are important. Some will be the same for everyone, such as health, family, and finances, but others will not. Parents may have different dimensions of their life than non-parents. Men may have different dimensions than women.

It doesn't matter. What matters is that each person consciously identifies, for themselves, all of the social dimensions of their life that are important to them. This refers to the social dimensions that, if missing, would leave a gaping hole in your quality of life—both now and in the future.

I first did this several years ago when I was on a plane returning home from a law conference. It was a time in my life when my level of health, happiness, and fulfillment weren't where I wanted them to be. They weren't where I knew they had to be in order for me to achieve the quality of life I desired.

As a corporate and commercial lawyer, many of my clients were business owners. Working with them, I got to see how (at least from the outside) exciting their lives appeared. Some of them owned or controlled businesses in different industries, or had multiple divisions within their main business. For example, one client I worked with had real estate, restaurant, and car wash businesses in his corporate stable. Another business owner I knew ran investment, immigration, golf course development, and software companies. At the time, I didn't have ownership interests in any businesses, and I was kind of bummed out that I didn't.

So, for whatever reason, on that flight home from the law conference I had the idea to treat my *life* as my own little corporate empire. I decided to sketch out all of the divisions of my life that were important to me and in which I knew I had to achieve success in order to experience the lasting health, happiness, and fulfillment that I longed for. Being a business lawyer, I decided to lay out my life as a corporate chart, with each division being an important aspect of my life. I didn't call them social dimensions then, but that's what they were. I called my fictitious corporate empire Andy Clark's Life Co. (ACL Co. for short) and, over time, I built it out with subdivisions in each dimension. And as I learned more about the concept of wellness and degrees of health and vitality, I realized that what I really wanted was to achieve a high degree of wellness in each of these dimensions. So I added the concept of wellness to each division, and called the whole thing my corporate wellness chart. A copy of it is reproduced on the next page, and I would encourage you to create your own.

ACL Co. Corporate Wellness Chart

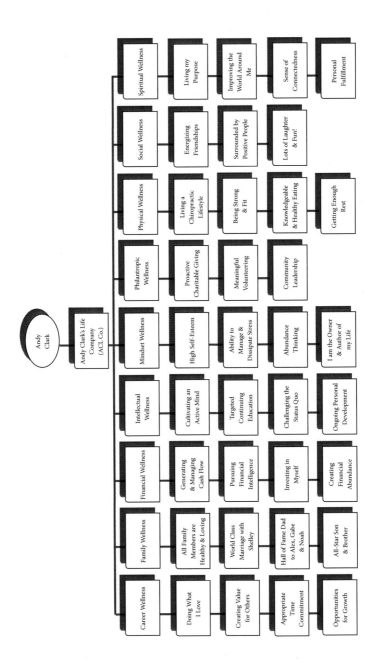

Andy Clark

Andy Clark's Life Company (ACL Co.)

Career Wellness
- Doing What I Love
- Creating Value for Others
- Appropriate Time Commitment
- Opportunities for Growth

Family Wellness
- All Family Members are Healthy & Loving
- World Class Marriage with Shelley
- Hall of Fame Dad to Alex, Gabe & Noah
- All-Star Son & Brother

Financial Wellness
- Generating & Managing Cash Flow
- Pursuing Financial Intelligence
- Investing in Myself
- Creating Financial Abundance

Intellectual Wellness
- Cultivating an Active Mind
- Targeted Continuing Education
- Challenging the Status Quo
- Ongoing Personal Development

Mindset Wellness
- High Self-Esteem
- Ability to Manage & Dissipate Stress
- Abundance Thinking
- I am the Owner & Author of my Life

Philantropic Wellness
- Proactive Charitable Giving
- Meaningful Volunteering
- Community Leadership

Physical Wellness
- Living a Chiropractic Lifestyle
- Being Strong & Fit
- Knowledgeable & Healthy Eating
- Getting Enough Rest

Social Wellness
- Energizing Friendships
- Surrounded by Positive People
- Lots of Laughter & Fun!

Spiritual Wellness
- Living my Purpose
- Improving the World Around Me
- Sense of Connectedness
- Personal Fulfillment

This experience was a game-changer for me. Getting conscious about all of the dimensions of my life to which I needed to devote time, energy, and resources (even if I wasn't currently doing so) was critical in helping me to achieve the vastly increased degree of wellness and quality of life that I enjoy today.

One major benefit I experienced as a result of creating my corporate wellness chart—especially as I became more knowledgeable about the concept of wellness—was the realization that two of the three physiological dimensions of wellness (physical and biochemical) were combined together in one of my social dimensions (physical wellness). The same will likely occur when you create your corporate wellness chart. In other words, your fitness and diet will probably be in *one* of your social dimensions. All of your other social dimensions of life (eight others, in my case) will relate to the psychological dimension of life, impacting how you think.

Take the financial dimension, for example. You can't eat money and it can't give you shelter from the elements. But having money can allow you to buy food and shelter. And *not* having money can impact your thoughts and actions and lead to negative psychological stress. And as we have discussed, a level of negative psychological stress that exceeds your GAP will eventually lead to illness or disease.

That's why, when looking for your starting point to improve the degree of wellness in your life, you must start with the psychological dimension of your life—how you think and what you think about. In terms of the social dimensions of your life, some of you will need to focus on your health and fitness first, some will need to look first at how to improve your career, and some of you will need to spend time and energy on one or more relationships in your life. Still others will need to focus on something else first and foremost.

But if we look at the physiological dimensions of life, there's no question that the place to start is the psychological dimension, since the vast majority of your social dimensions relate to the psychological dimension of your life. Sure, exercising (physical) and eating right (biochemical) have a huge impact on your ability to think clearly and positively, and on your ability to dissipate mental stress. That can't be overstated. But equally true is that the *choice* to exercise and eat right in the first place is directed by your thoughts. Whether consciously or subconsciously, it all starts in your mind. Thoughts become things.

You can look at it this way. Quality of life is determined by your degree of health and vitality. Your degree of health and vitality is determined by your lifestyle. Your lifestyle is determined by your daily choices and actions. And those choices and actions are determined by your thoughts. It all starts with your thoughts—how you think, what you think about, and the level of consciousness you bring to your life. So, when seeking to improve your degree of wellness and the quality of your life, look first to the psychological dimension of life. In the next chapter, you'll discover why lawyers are perfectly positioned to do just that.

5

WHY LAWYERS ARE PERFECTLY POSITIONED TO ADOPT A WELLNESS LIFESTYLE

It's so easy to make excuses to avoid adopting a wellness lifestyle—especially for lawyers. For starters, it's not an easy thing to do. It requires a significant amount of self-discipline, planning, dedication, and commitment. And lawyers more than most people have little time to allocate to all of the important dimensions of their lives. Practicing law seems to suck up the vast majority of your time, and there's just not a whole lot left over to invest in health, friends, family, and community. It's not that we're bad people; it's not that we don't want to operate at a high level in every important area of our lives. It's just that we're so damn busy all the time.

Plus, you will recall Dr. Seligman's line of thinking that the same personality trait that makes us good lawyers—pessimism— also tends to make us unhappy people. The theory goes that the practice of law attracts pessimists and then the continued practice of law entrenches that pessimism (and unhappiness) year after year.

So you don't have to work too hard to build a case strong enough to justify that the practice of law and wellness cannot co-exist—that the term lawyer wellness is an oxymoron. As with most anything in life, you can see what you want to see. You can blame your clients, or your partners, or your firm, or the profession if you experience any of the 3 Uns, and you'll find plenty of support for your position: Misery loves company, after all.

But if you've made it this far into this book, you're probably not one of those lawyers. If so, here's some great news for you: Lawyers are perfectly positioned to successfully and sustainably adopt the wellness lifestyle required to experience lasting health, happiness, and fulfillment. While there's some truth to all of the reasons you can espouse *not* to adopt a wellness lifestyle, you don't need to let them determine the quality of your life. You are the author of your own life; you control your own destiny. You decide if you're going to suffer the perpetual pain of one or more of the 3 Uns in your life because it's too hard not to, or you don't have enough self-discipline, or you don't have enough time. But just know this: Being unhealthy, unhappy, or unfulfilled for a good portion of your life—to me, *that* is hard. By comparison, doing the things required to live a wellness lifestyle, and thus to experience lasting health, happiness, and fulfillment, to me, that is a hell of a lot easier and a hell of a lot smarter. And more fun, too.

Dr. Seligman may have a point when he says that pessimism makes us good lawyers, but unhappy people. But why do we need to focus on that? Why not focus on some other essential characteristics of being a good lawyer that *also* can be employed to get us well and keep us well so that we *can* experience lasting health, happiness, and fulfillment. There are plenty of them to choose from, and in this chapter I'll focus on three: logical reasoning, consciousness, and integrity. Each of these skills is required not just to be a good lawyer, but to be a lawyer at all. If you're a lawyer, you have these skills in spades; you just may not have learned to apply them to your personal life in a manner that would enhance your degree of health and vitality. You're about to learn that now.

Let's look at each of these skillsets in turn.

LOGICAL REASONING

Above all else, lawyers are practitioners of logic. We don't even get into law school without showing an aptitude for logical reasoning; it is a central component of the LSAT. Dictionary definitions of logic include theory or system of reasoning; sensible argument and thought; and relationship and pattern of events. This is what we are trained to do as lawyers, and this is what we do every day. We are paid to bring sensible argument and thought to a particular set of circumstances, to see the relationship and pattern of events, and to apply a theory or system of reasoning to those circumstances and events in order to advocate for the result our clients desire. The best lawyers aren't just practitioners of logic—they're sorcerers of logic. They use logic in such a way that even opposing counsel end up agreeing with their view, since if they did not they would be seen to be arguing with plain logic.

So it's lawyers more than anyone who have the skillset to allow them to understand and apply the Law of Cause and Effect in their lives. Lawyers get the logic that the effects we see in our lives are the results of the causes we have created with our past choices and actions. Lawyers, more than most, can appreciate the logic that health, happiness, and fulfillment are critical to our quantity and quality of life, and that in order to experience those things in a sustained way throughout our lives we must live a wellness lifestyle, a manner of living that enhances our degree of health and vitality. And as will be discussed below, lawyers understand the perfect logic that this manner of living requires choices and actions that are congruent with their most important values, and with the degree of wellness they want to experience in each dimension of their lives.

Lawyers have the perfect logical skillset to see that the allopathic or sickness and treatment paradigm of health is perfectly illogical when applied to chronic illness. They can see the defects of a system that knows chronic illness is caused by lifestyle factors and not genetics, but mostly ignores that fact when diagnosing and treating illness. Whereas others may blindly follow men and women in white coats prescribing white pills for illnesses caused by a toxic or deficient cellular environment, lawyers are hard wired to question and not take things for granted just because that's the paradigm most people follow. We're not most people. We're trained and paid to offer new perspectives and to appreciate the logical positions put forth by others. We're also trained and paid to spot illogical arguments and, with the use of logic, to systematically break them down to demonstrate their failure to abide by the Law of Cause and Effect.

Lawyers also know the importance of questions. We need to ask the right questions of our clients to figure out what the issues are and how we can help them. We need to ask the right questions on discovery or deposition to get the facts on which to base our legal arguments. We need to ask the right questions of witnesses at trial to elicit the evidence required to prove our case. So we are well versed and skilled in the art of questions, and we can appreciate the crucial importance of asking the right questions.

RCTs: The question is everything

Let's look at this further by exploring the concept of randomized controlled trials (RCTs). RCTs have become the gold standard of evidence-based scientific research. RCTs are used to prove the efficacy and relative safety of a healthcare intervention—most often a pharmaceutical drug. In the views of many in the allopathic paradigm, an intervention that does not have several RCTs to back it up is not evidence-based and should not be approved for use.

In an RCT, participants meeting desired criteria (for example, they exhibit symptoms of a certain health condition) are divided into groups randomly. One group receives the intervention that is the subject of the trial (a new drug), another group receives a placebo, and in some cases a third group receives nothing at all. If at the conclusion of the trial, it is shown that the intervention was more successful at removing the symptoms of the health condition than the placebo (or doing nothing at all), while meeting safety standards, the trial is deemed successful. Generally, two successful trials are required before an intervention can be approved for use in the general population. That all appears to make good sense.

But here's where the question becomes paramount. Dr. Chestnut illustrates the point by supposing there was an RCT of wilting plants.[61] Half the plants are given water and the other half are given fake water. The allopathic model asks this question: Does water reduce or remove the wilting? In the hypothetical trial, none of the plants showed a reduction in wilting after ten weeks. The allopathic conclusion is that water does not help plants wilt less, and therefore water is no good for wilting plants. Anyone that gives wilting plants water is not practicing evidence-based gardening.

But what if the question is this: Did the plants that received water become healthier than the plants that did not? Well, we know that plants need water, so yes, the plants that received water for ten weeks are healthier than the plants that received no water—regardless of whether they were still wilting. Based on that question, we can conclude that water is good for wilting plants.

Same plants, same trial, diametrically opposed conclusions. The first says water is no good for wilting plants. The second says it is. The second might consider that the cause of the wilting wasn't lack of water; perhaps it was lack of sunlight, or lack of nutrients in the soil, or too much toxicity in the soil. But just because the plants didn't stop wilting did not mean that water isn't good for wilting plants.

Dr. Chestnut's plant analogy illustrates the limitations of symptom-based interventions and the RCT as the gold standard of evidence-based healthcare. It seems so obvious. You don't even need to have the smarts of a lawyer to figure it out. Yet in most industrialized nations, this is the system we are living in—a paradigm based on faulty logic and the wrong questions.

This is yet another way in which lawyers can be leaders in shaping the paradigm shift towards a wellness and prevention model and away from the sickness and treatment model that dominates today. A successful health care model isn't more sick people accessing properly prescribed drugs; it is fewer sick people in the first place. And to have achieve that, people need to do the things that are known to produce health and vitality: consume a plant-based, whole foods diet; exercise daily; get ample rest; reduce levels of mental and emotional stress; enhance feelings of love, gratitude, and connectedness; and so on. We'll look at each of these things and more in the next two chapters.

As lawyers, we understand that emotion is an essential part of life, and we do not disregard the presence and importance of emotion in our work, but above all we live in and promote a world governed by logic and reason. Therefore, when we see the commercial about the guy suffering from heartburn after eating a plate of fried, greasy food, we think maybe the guy should eat less fried, greasy food so that he wouldn't get heartburn, rather than what the advertiser wants us to think, which is to take more Zantac so you can go on eating fried, greasy food. The crazy thing is, taking pills for this, that, and the other thing has become so commonplace in our society that most people will watch that commercial without even thinking twice about how ridiculous it is. *Bad lifestyle choices making me sick? No problem! I'll pop a few pills so I can go on making bad lifestyle choices!*

But as lawyers, we're able to spot the lunacy in the world around us and we're well positioned to do something about it. We are agents of change—or at least we should be. And a great place to start, in the words of Patrick Schiltz, is to stop stampeding like buffalo and to begin to think more logically about why we're leading the lives we're leading. That's the focus of the next section.

CONSCIOUSNESS

Consciousness means awareness of a particular issue and of your surroundings. When applied to wellness, consciousness means actively steering your life in the direction you choose. It's choosing to live your life by design rather than by default. It requires identifying all of the areas of your life that are important to you and figuring out what you want in each area. As part of this process, your core values will emerge, since you value those things that are important to you.

When you do this—when you live consciously—you give yourself the gift of a decision-making framework. This is not to be underestimated. Most lawyers do not have a consciously developed and fully formed decision-making framework to guide their lives. This makes life hard—and makes us unwell.

When you don't know with clarity where you're going in your life, where you want to end up, what is important to you and what you value, then every decision you make in the run of a day requires a significant investment of energy and adds unnecessary stress to your life.

What time will I get up in the morning? What will I have for breakfast? Will I exercise? When? For how long? Should I buy this? Can I afford that? How long should I work today? What should I work on? Do I have time for lunch? Should I call my mother today? Should I make it home for dinner? What will I have for dinner? Should I go to that event next week? Should I let my teenager go to that party? Should I join the board of that non-profit? Should I? Can I? Will I?

Without a fully formed decision-making framework, you can't confidently identify what opportunities you should pursue. Often you can't even spot opportunities in the first place. Worse, you might mistake obstacles for opportunities, and vice versa.

When you have a conscious and clear vision of what you want and where you want to go in your life, these decisions become much easier. Will this move me closer down the path that I have set out for myself? Yes? Then I'll do it. No? Then I won't. The amount of energy this saves, and the amount of unnecessary stress this reduces in your life is significant on a daily basis—and it is exponentially significant over the course of a lifetime. And since energy and stress are key determinants of your overall level of wellness, anything you can do to increase the former and decrease the latter leads to better short-term and long-term health.

Take sports for example. I played a lot of hockey growing up and in college. When you play hockey you need to keep your head up, so that you can spot the open teammate and avoid an opponent's bodycheck. If your head's down, you miss both the opportunity to improve your position and you put yourself in harm's way. Many lawyers would be well-served by keeping their heads up more often, and this is much easier to do once you've given yourself a decision-making framework to help guide you.

If sports analogies don't do it for you, think back to the dehydrated, dying lawyer in the desert from Chapter 3. He was so focused on water that he didn't give any thought as to why not one but two nomads offered him a necktie in the middle of the desert. He mistook the nomads as obstacles rather than opportunities. Of course, it's tough to blame him. I've never been close to death from dehydration, but I imagine it's pretty hard to think clearly in that state. But many well-hydrated lawyers fail to think clearly across all dimensions of their life—again, because they lack a decision-making framework that comes with an enhanced degree of consciousness applied to each dimension.

Consciousness requires thinking and paying attention. These are things we do all day at work, but as a group we don't do as well away from the office. There may be lots of good reasons for this, not the least of which is that we may want or need a break from thinking when we transition into our personal lives after using our brains in a concerted way for hours on end at work every day. But if you want health, happiness, and fulfillment in your life—and if you're reading this book, then you probably do—then you simply can't afford to stop thinking when you're not on the clock at work. Just as the separation of work and life is illogical when applied to the concept of work-life balance, it is also illogical to turn off your brain when you're not working; you need to bring the same level of thinking and consciousness to your whole life as you bring to the practice of law. You need to sit down and think logically about the life you are leading; you need to identify your top values and think through what you want in each dimension of life; and you need to apply values-based decision-making to your entire life. If you fail to do this, that will cause the effect of experiencing one or more of the 3Uns in a sustained manner throughout your life. It will erode your quality of life and will cause you to violate another of the key characteristics you require to practice law: integrity.

INTEGRITY

Integrity is revealed when your actions and choices are congruent with your vision and values. Nathaniel Branden, the leading authority on the science of self-esteem, defines it this way: "Integrity is the integration of ideals, convictions, standards, beliefs—and behavior. When our behavior is congruent with our professed values, when ideals and practice match up, we have integrity."[62] In other words, integrity means doing what you say you're going to do.

Our ethical obligations as lawyers compel us to act with integrity professionally—to do what we say we're going to do. Lawyers who have incongruence between their professional words and actions don't last very long in this business—at best they have a sullied reputation, and at worst they get disbarred. Yet while most lawyers are clear on how integrity impacts their law practice, many fail to fully appreciate the foundational role integrity plays in the rest of their lives. Lack of congruence in your life is a massive destroyer of wellness, because it leads to energy leakage and stress.

Incongruence can be conscious: *Sam, I know I said I'd meet you at 3:00, but I've got to get this other thing done, so I'm not going to be able to make it.* You said you were going to do something (meet Sam at 3:00) but you're not going to do it—and whether that's due to circumstances within or outside of your control doesn't much matter. An incongruence—a lack of integrity—between what you said you were going to do and what you actually did has occurred. Not a big deal as an isolated incident—Sam will most likely understand if it's the first time—but these can add up over time. Try this a few times and you'll find that Sam isn't as interested in making plans to meet you anymore.

I should mention that incongruence and lack of integrity also consciously occur when people lie, cheat, and steal. People like that certainly lack integrity, but they don't have any sense of morality or judgment either, and this book doesn't claim to or intend to provide help or guidance for people like that. This book, and in particular this chapter, is about the good, honest people, as the vast majority of lawyers are, who unknowingly fail to incorporate an appropriate level of integrity into their overall lives.

Most incongruence in our lives is subconscious and thus more insidious—we aren't even aware of its existence. For example, you may have identified health as a top core value, as one of the most important areas of your life. *I deeply value my health,* you might say. But do your actions support that? Do you *do* the things that are congruent with valuing your health? Do you exercise, eat well, get enough rest, manage your professional stress, and limit other negative stressors in your life? If you don't, then you have a massive incongruence in your life—a lack of integrity—that erodes your health big time.

This is a fairly obvious—and common—example of incongruence in many lawyers' lives, and it's easy to draw the line between this example and a resulting lack of health and vitality.

But there are other examples of incongruence in many lawyers' lives that can be equally damaging to their wellness unbeknownst to them. If you have identified family as an important area of your life—as a top core value—but you're not investing the requisite time and energy into supporting that core value, then you have a major incongruence in your life. Are you spending enough quality time with your spouse and kids? Are you present and attentive during that time? Do you communicate with your family members with love, respect, and compassion, or does pettiness, resentment, jealousy, or anger creep into those communications?

You may also have money as a core value, and you may have identified financial wellness as a key component of your ideal life. But do your actions support that? Do you work hard enough and smart enough to create the financial abundance you seek? Do you create a lot of value for others, or do you have some sense of entitlement that money should just flow to you as some sort of right?

When it comes to core values and what's important to lawyers, there are no inherently right or wrong answers. What *is* right or wrong, however, is whether or not your actions are congruent with those values. Some lawyers may need to work and bill more to achieve congruence in their lives. Others may need to work and bill less. Some may need to do different work altogether. There is no one-size-fits-all approach here.

What *is* universal, however, is that congruence with consciously identified values—living with integrity—is energy producing, stress reducing, and health promoting. A lack of congruence and integrity has just the opposite effect and will negatively impact the degree of health and vitality you experience in your life.

Lawyers who apply logic, consciousness, and integrity in their professional and personal lives will achieve a high level of overall wellness and a tremendous quality of life. Lawyers who don't, won't. It's as simple as that. Of course, this applies only to lawyers who place a high priority on short- and long-term health and vitality in their lives. That is to say that experiencing a high degree of health and vitality is one of their top core values; they are conscious about the importance of health and vitality in their lives, and they act with integrity with that value. If you're reading a book about lawyer wellness, then it's a safe bet that your health and vitality are pretty important to you.

As a profession, we need to start applying to our personal lives the amount of logic, consciousness, and integrity that we bring to our professional lives. The framework and skillset is already there. If lawyers can apply logic, consciousness, and integrity to our overall lives, we'll be able to transform the perception and reality of practicing law from "unwellness" to wellness. What a precedent to set for the rest of the world.

CONSCIOUSNESS, INTEGRITY, AND HABITS

A habit is a regularly repeated behavior pattern. As we all know, habits can be positive or negative, good or bad, healthy or unhealthy. Often our habits go unnoticed in our lives because we are not conscious about them. Every time we repeat our habits, they lead our lives in a certain direction. The question is, where are your habits leading you?

Before you can begin to answer that question, you need to figure out what your habits are in the first place. Just as with identifying your core values, identifying your habits requires bringing a high level of consciousness to your life. It requires paying attention to and noticing all of the things you do every day—especially the things you're in the habit of doing automatically. Then you can decide whether those habits are leading you in the life direction you want, or whether they are steering you off course. Most likely, some of your habits will be supporting your life's ambitions, and others will be undermining them.

A key ingredient in a wellness lifestyle is to create wellness habits that become engrained and are a part of who you are. It's not easy, but in the long run, the alternative will be much, much harder. Do you want your life to be a little bit easy now and a lot harder later, or a little bit hard now and a lot easier later? As Jim Rohn said, "we must all suffer one of two things: The pain of discipline or the pain of regret." Which would you prefer?

Bob Bowman, coach of Olympic champion American swimmer Michael Phelps, said "successful people make a habit of doing things other people aren't willing to do." It's a great quote. I like it even better when you replace the concept of success with the concept of health, like this: *Healthy people make a habit of doing things other people aren't willing to do.*

Make it a habit to exercise for 30 minutes a day. Make it a habit to express gratitude for all that you have on a daily basis. Make it a habit to drive by (not through) fast food restaurants. Make it a habit to have weekly date nights with your spouse. Make it a habit to be around positive people—and to avoid negative people.

The list goes on. But the good thing is, you don't have to change your whole life at once. Start small. Make only one change at a time. You just need to get the ball rolling and then momentum takes over. Start with baby steps, and you'll be shocked at just how much of an impact small changes can make in your life and how quickly you can turn them into positive, permanent habits.

If you're concerned that you don't have the self-discipline to create wellness habits, consider this: We're all 100% self-disciplined to our current habits. The missing ingredient isn't self-discipline; it's establishing the right habits. It's not change that we fear; it's transition to change—that is the hard part. Bad habits die hard and new ones can be difficult to implement. Common wisdom says that it takes between 21 and 30 days to create a new habit, and that has proved correct in my experience. You have to have considerable resolve and dedication to create a new habit. But transition to change doesn't last a lifetime. It lasts three to four weeks—that's less than a month. Once the habit is created, then you can switch back to autopilot with respect to that habit; it becomes part of who you are. You no longer have to expend the mental energy to decide if you're going to do something, you just do it because it's a habit. If you have a young child, do you have to think about whether or not you're going to buckle that child into a car seat before you begin driving? Of course not, it's just something you do every single time. As Jack Canfield of *Chicken Soup for the Soul* fame said, "99% is a bitch, 100% is a breeze."

So it's the transition of breaking habits that don't serve us, and creating ones that do, that is the hard part. In order to succeed in this transition phase, your purpose for creating wellness habits must be stronger than the obstacles that will present themselves to derail your best-laid plans. At times, the world seems to conspire against us in our attempts to live a wellness lifestyle. Not only does your career as a lawyer—with its long hours and high-stress environments—make consistent wellness practice a challenge, but the barrage of media promoting pharmaceuticals, alcohol, fast food, and other wellness undermining products can be tough to fight off, too. In addition, the sheer volume of information we are deluged by on a daily basis—of a legal and non-legal nature—is enough to cause stress and overwhelm us on its own.

These forces of media, technology, and information overload aren't going away any time soon, but if you apply the 6Cs of Wellness, you'll set yourself up for success on your journey towards greater health, happiness, and fulfillment in your life.

THE 6CS OF WELLNESS

Your transition to a wellness lifestyle will require a growing understanding and mastery of the 6Cs of Wellness: control, consciousness, creativity, clarity, certainty and congruence.

> ➤ *Control* refers to the idea that you are the author of your life. The degree to which you experience health and vitality in your life is the result of your choices and actions—your lifestyle—and you control your choices and actions. No one else is pulling your puppet strings. Take responsibility for the outcome of your life by owning the idea that you are in control of it.
>
> ➤ *Consciousness*, as discussed, is thinking deeply about all aspects of your life. It's thinking logically about why you're leading the life you're leading. It's identifying what you want in all of the important dimensions of your life and assessing whether or not your daily choices, actions, and habits get you closer to achieving what you want, or take you further away from it.
>
> ➤ *Creativity* means that the clearest path to wellness may not be the most obvious one. You may need to think about things a little differently than you have in the past in order to overcome obstacles and to achieve your desired outcome. Great lawyers are creative problem solvers. Michael Melcher wrote an entire book about this called

The Creative Lawyer, in which he writes that a "creative lawyer is any lawyer who uses his or her own creativity to make a life that works."[63] Einstein's great quote is also relevant here: "The definition of insanity is doing the same thing over and over and expecting different results."

➤ *Clarity* is the degree to which you are conscious. It's knowing *exactly* what you want and what you need to do to get it. The more clarity you bring to your life, the more likely you are to achieve what you want. Fuzzy targets don't get hit.

➤ *Certainty* is an absolute conviction in your beliefs. It's believing without a doubt in what you want and your ability to achieve it. There will be lots of doubters and naysayers on your road to a wellness lifestyle, and your degree of certainty will determine if those doubters and naysayers derail your efforts, provide a minor road bump, or aren't even noticed at all. Certainty trumps doubt every time.

➤ *Congruence*, as discussed, means acting in accordance with your consciously defined values. It's doing what you say you're going to do. It's being and living in integrity and applying values-based decision making across all dimensions of your life.

The degree to which you master these 6Cs of Wellness will play a large part in determining the degree to which you experience health and vitality in your life.

In the next two chapters, I will cover some specific strategies and best practices that lawyers can apply in each dimension of their lives. Before moving on, however, I want to share this passage with you from *The Lawyer Bubble*: "Those who attribute the current state of the legal profession to market forces beyond anyone's control are wrong. Human decisions created this mess; better human decisions can clean it up."[64]

The same holds true for your current levels of health, happiness, and fulfillment. These are the result of your decisions, and if they are a mess, better decisions can clean them up.

6

BEST PRACTICES IN THE
PHYSIOLOGICAL DIMENSIONS OF LIFE

What does a wellness lifestyle look like in practice? What are the nuts and bolts of a manner of living that enhances health and vitality in all dimensions of life? Because we're all different, and we're starting from different places in the wellness continuum and at different stages of life, and because we'll all have some different social dimensions of life that may need more attention than others, it stands to reason that your wellness lifestyle may look different than mine or anyone else's. Nevertheless, there will be common ingredients in everyone's recipe for wellness, and other ingredients that will appear in the recipes of most. In this chapter, I'll describe some best practices in each of the physiological dimensions of life. In the next chapter, I'll cover some best practices in the social dimensions of life that are common to most lawyers.

Let's take a moment to refresh as to the key benefits you'll experience as a result of incorporating these best practices into your lifestyle.

Key benefits of a wellness lifestyle

- ➢ Enhanced health
- ➢ Enhanced happiness
- ➢ Enhanced fulfillment

Enhanced quantity and quality of life

> ➤ You'll think better
> ➤ You'll have more energy
> ➤ You'll experience less stress
> ➤ You'll gain enhanced confidence
> ➤ You'll enjoy a greater sense of control
> ➤ You'll develop a clearer sense of purpose

Increased
effectiveness
as a lawyer

Not a bad list, is it? Any one of these benefits might be reason enough to finally and permanently adopt a wellness lifestyle, but you don't have to settle for just one. If you take ownership of your career and your overall life like you have never done before—if you take complete responsibility for the outcome of your experience on this Earth, and you decide once and for all to take control of your health, happiness, and fulfillment—you will experience *all* of these benefits. Not maybe. Not probably. You *will*. The Law of Cause and Effect guarantees it.

I make no representation that this chapter and the next contain an exhaustive list of wellness practices, or that the practices that are included in these chapters are covered in the depth that they deserve. Entire libraries have been written about each of the practices discussed in the pages that follow. My purpose in these next two chapters is to give you a taste of some of the best practices in each dimension of life that, if applied, will move you further to the right of the wellness continuum. Some of these practices you might have considered before, and others you might not have. I encourage you to learn more about these practices over the months and years ahead. Remember, self-responsibility means taking ownership over the outcome of your life; it's not something you can delegate.

Not every best practice described in Chapters 6 and 7 will deliver all of the above benefits to your life, but if you incorporate enough of the practices into your lifestyle, you will experience all of these benefits. Some of the practices described will resonate more with you than others; some you may have already mastered, others you may be struggling to adopt, and still others you may swear you'll never do in a hundred years. That's all fine. As mentioned, your wellness lifestyle will look a little different in practice than most everyone else's. But I encourage you to at least try each of the practices discussed—even the ones that scare the heck out of you. Those are the ones that may end up increasing your overall degree of health and vitality the most.

Remember when reading these next two chapters that the boundaries between dimensions of life are fluid, not rigid. Each of the practices discussed has been listed under a specific dimension of your life—either in the physiological or social category—but many of these will benefit you in other dimensions as well. A win in *any* dimension of life is a win in *every* dimension of life.

It is important for you to realize when reading through these best practices that you don't need to adopt them all at once—that would be a recipe for failure. It's best to proceed one at a time. Pick one practice that you think will be a high leverage point for you in terms of catapulting your degree of health and vitality forward, and make a goal to turn that practice into a habit. As discussed in the last chapter, it will take 21 to 30 days to turn a new practice into a habit—but once you do, the practice will become part of your lifestyle, and you won't have to expend much energy to think about it anymore. It will just be something that you do; it'll be part of *who you are.*

If you turn one of these practices into a habit every month for the next year, you'll have incorporated 12 new habits into your lifestyle by the time the calendar flips back around. Just think about the massive leap forward that will mean to the degree of health and vitality you'll experience across all dimensions of your life. I guarantee that will significantly enhance your effectiveness as a lawyer *and* your overall quality of life. And the best part is that you can proceed in baby steps— one best practice at a time—so that you won't get overwhelmed trying to make too many changes at once. The purpose of a wellness lifestyle is to decrease stress in your life, not add more of it! Plus, proceeding slowly with one practice at a time will make your journey to increased health and vitality more sustainable, enjoyable, and fun.

Let's get started.

PHYSICAL WELLNESS

You will recall from Chapter 4 that the physical dimension of life, as it relates to the physiological dimensions, is about what you do (or don't do) with your body. It's about how much exercise you get; it's about your quality and quantity of sleep; it's about your posture and how much sitting you do each day, and other ways your physical body moves or doesn't move. Physical wellness also includes the absence of trauma—broken legs, concussions, flesh wounds, etc.—but I won't focus on the prevention of trauma here. For the most part, physical trauma occurs by accident—it's often preventable, yes, but still accidental. Here, I'll focus on the primary driver of physical wellness over which you, and only you, have complete control: Exercise.

Exercise

The benefits of exercise are many. Here are just a few of them:

Exercise makes you healthier: There's a long list of illnesses and diseases that exercise has been shown to help prevent: arthritis, Alzheimer's, diabetes, heart disease, cancer, anxiety, depression, and so on. One study found that a low fitness level was the strongest predictor of death among all risk factors studied.[65] That is all great and worth knowing, but it is an allopathic view of the benefits of exercise. In the wellness and prevention paradigm, you don't have to study particular diseases to see if exercise is beneficial or not. The premise is much simpler: Our genetic blueprint *requires* exercise in order to express health. Yes, exercise prevents illness and disease. But even more important, exercise increases health and vitality. Regular exercise is an essential ingredient that our cells require in order to express health.

Exercise reduces negative stress: What lawyer wouldn't love to have a little less stress in their life? Regular physical activity helps you process and dissipate negative stress more effectively. Researchers have discovered that exercise "does nothing less than reshape your brain, making it more stress-resistant" and that "the positive stress of exercise prepares structures and pathways within the brain so that they're more equipped to handle stress in other forms."[66]

Exercise makes you think better: Research shows that when you're under a lot of stress, you don't think as well. And since thinking is what lawyers are paid to do, the better you think, the better you do your job, and the more value you deliver to your clients. So when you're under a lot of stress, you don't do what you're paid to do as well as you should. Consequently, when you exercise regularly, thereby reducing your levels of negative stress, you'll think more clearly.

Exercise helps you sleep better: Exercise helps you sleep better, and we all know what a difference being well-rested makes when practicing law (not to mention how we deal with our children and handle our emotions).

Exercise gives you more energy: To those who are new to regular exercise, it may seem counterintuitive, but exercise doesn't deplete your energy stores; on the contrary, it gives you *more* energy. Ask any colleague who exercises regularly and they'll confirm that for you. That's why a mid-day workout can be so beneficial: It gives you the boost of energy you may need to combat the post-lunch fatigue that many lawyers experience. I have started many workouts feeling somewhat lethargic only to finish exercising 30 minutes later with a newfound energy. Einstein said that compound interest is the eighth wonder of the world. I disagree—I think it's the energy-producing effects of exercise.

Exercise makes you happier: Exercise has been found to lower depression, so there's a good chance that working out regularly will make you happier, too. As Harvard's Tal Ben-Shahar has noted, "not exercising is like taking a depressant."[67]

How much exercise do you need?

How much exercise do you need to experience these benefits? The consensus appears to be 30 minutes a day of moderate exercise. If you haven't seen it yet, you should check out the visual lecture that Canadian M.D. Mike Evans posted on YouTube about the massive benefits of exercise. It's called *23 ½ hours: what is the single best thing we can do for our health?*[68] In the video, Dr. Evans describes the laundry list of benefits that a particular "intervention" has been shown to create (including many of the benefits listed above). He leads the viewer to believe that the intervention is yet another pharmaceutical, but finally discloses that the wonder drug is exercise, the appropriate dose of which is about 30 minutes of walking daily.

For those new to exercise, 30 minutes of walking daily is certainly a good start. But to achieve a higher level of physical fitness, you will need to increase the intensity over time. The good news is that when you increase the intensity of the exercise—by running or trying cross-training like a cardio/strength training blend—you can decrease the length of your workout. The best results I have ever seen in my physical fitness have resulted from high intensity 15 to 20 minute workouts five or six days a week.

I know you're busy, but are you *really* too busy to find 20 to 30 minutes per day to exercise, given all of the benefits that you'll experience, and all of the illness and disease that you're likely to avoid as a result?

A common misconception among lawyers is that you need to go to a gym to exercise. You don't. Your firm may pay for or subsidize a gym membership—which is wonderful, and you should take advantage of it—but don't hang out with the "I don't have time to get to the gym" crowd. It's not about going to the gym. If you don't have time to get to the gym, then go for a walk or a jog, or get a workout DVD—there are plenty of great ones on the market that will run you through a full body workout in 20 or 30 minutes. There is an article in the Best of the Blog section of this book about just how much time you can save by exercising this way, without sacrificing the quality of your workout. Indeed, it's probably better than a longer workout at the gym.

If you're really time-crunched and you can't find 20 minutes in the day to exercise, try to find 10, or even five. Do some jumping jacks or pushups, or jog on the spot just to get your heart rate going a little bit. That alone will recharge a tired mind and will make you a more effective lawyer for the hour or two that follows. A little exercise is better than none, no matter how little. Or consider using exercise as your mode of transportation to and from work. Matthew Latella, a partner in Baker & McKenzie's Toronto office, has been riding his bicycle to work most days for the better part of 10 years. While he certainly isn't the only lawyer who uses pedal power for his daily commute, he says his chosen method of commuting still seems novel. "I use the shower facilities at the office complex where I work, and, despite there being only two shower stalls available for all the men working in approximately 100 stories of office space, in all the years I've been biking to work I have never had to wait to use the showers."

What's the best time of day to exercise? That would be whenever you're most likely to do it. I think it's best to exercise first thing in the morning, so that it's done and out of the way and no one can take it away from you no matter how they might try at the office later that day. But that may not work for everyone. Some prefer a mid-afternoon workout to re-energize after lunch when the mind starts to fatigue. Others prefer to workout at night with their spouse after the kids are in bed. Whatever works best for you is the best time for you to work out. If you'd like to be a morning exerciser, but you just aren't a morning person, check out the article "10-steps to start your day with exercise" that appears in the Best of the Blog section of the book.

Whatever time you pick for your workouts, an unequivocal best practice is to time block your exercise. Diana Richmond, partner at Richmond, Chickloski, Igras, Moldowan in Calgary explains: "Take that hour to workout no matter what. Just organize the rest of your day around it. Make it part of your calendar. It should be just as important as a client appointment or a court date. I schedule around my workouts. Selfish? Maybe, but it's what works for me." Maurice Chiasson, a partner in Stewart McKelvey's Halifax office, agrees. "The important part everyone needs to realize," he says, "is that fitness, like any other commitment, needs to be part of one's daily schedule. You need to make time for it like any other meeting or client commitment." Chiasson used this strategy to lose close to 100 pounds over the last few years. You can read more about his incredible story in the Best of the Blog section of the book.

Hiring a personal trainer is a great way to kick start your physical wellness, especially if you need some accountability to make sure you follow through on your exercise commitments. Not only are they knowledgeable about physiology and can put you on a program designed just for you, there's something about standing someone up—especially someone to whom you're paying good money—that will dramatically increase the odds of getting your butt out of bed in the morning to work out.

Working out at set times with friends is a way to build accountability into the equation without the added cost of a personal trainer—and it makes exercising a lot more fun too. If you're hanging out with people who don't want to work out, then join a class—yoga, spin, CrossFit, whatever—where you'll meet new people who can help hold you accountable.

In addition to exercise, you should also be mindful of how much sitting you're doing at the office and at home. Humans were not genetically designed to be as sedentary as most of us have become in modern times. Movement of any kind—even if it's not technically exercise—is good. Sitting for extended periods while hunched over a desk or cranking out a brief on your laptop is not. Take plenty of breaks while you're working. Get up and go for a 5-minute walk around the office every hour or so. And if you really want to ensure you get lots of movement throughout the day, consider a treadmill desk, so that you can work and move at the same time.

Chiropractic

In addition to exercise, another best practice in the physical dimension is to get adjusted regularly by a doctor of chiropractic. Many people have misconceptions about what chiropractors do, or they have no idea what chiropractors do at all. In short, doctors of chiropractic detect nerve interference caused by spinal misalignments, or subluxations, and they correct this nerve interference with chiropractic adjustments.

Negative stressors in the physiological dimensions of life cause subluxations, so chances are you have subluxations right now that are impeding optimal nerve flow throughout your body. This is a big deal, since everything that you experience or express in your life is processed through your nervous system—the master controller system of your body that detects signals from your internal and external environments. Therefore, your body's ability to process and dissipate stress, to self-heal and self-regulate, and to express health and vitality, will all be compromised to the degree of the nerve interference.

If you've never been assessed by a chiropractor, I would recommend that you do so. Look for a doctor who teaches patients about the manner in which stressors of modern living cause subluxation, and what you can do to reduce or eliminate those stressors.

BIOCHEMICAL WELLNESS

The biochemical dimension of life is what you put into (or don't put into) your body: food, drink, tobacco, drugs, vitamins, the air you breathe, the personal hygiene products you use, and so on. Simply put, there are good things you can put into your body, and there are bad things. With the possible exception of the air you breathe, you control whether most of the things you put into your body are good for you or not. As discussed in Chapter 3, we are genetically designed to express health, but we need the right building blocks to do so. One of the most important building blocks is proper nutrition; our cells require certain nutrients to function optimally.

Nutrition

On the surface—and mass media does its best to have you believe this—the subject of nutrition can be complicated. Today's news report might tell you to eat broccoli to reduce cancer risk, and tomorrow's might tell you to avoid broccoli to reduce cancer risk.

How can you make sense of it all? In truth, what to put in your body and what to avoid is a whole lot simpler than that, and I'll explain why in a moment. But first, let's look at why it's important to bother figuring it out. Let's look at the benefits of proper nutrition.

In many respects, the benefits of proper nutrition are the same as the benefits of exercise. Giving your cells the right nutrients to work with makes you think better and more clearly, gives you more energy, helps you sleep better, and gives you a better emotional balance.[69] All of these benefits cannot help but make you a more effective lawyer. And of course, a nutrient-rich diet will also help to extend your healthy lifespan, so that you'll have a much better chance of attending your granddaughter's wedding than you would consuming a nutrient-poor diet.

As with exercise, many research studies and media reports focus on what foods you should consume in order to decrease the likelihood of a particular illness. Eat this to avoid that. Eat that to avoid this. These studies all fall into the allopathic paradigm and should be viewed with caution. As Dr. James Chestnut notes, it is "an impossible task to identify every nutrient that cells require. We are discovering new essential nutrients all the time. The good news is that they are all in FOOD (whole foods). Of course they are. There is nothing that we need that is not provided from nature."[70]

The more sensible view—and the simpler view, as promised above—is to look at what our cells genetically require to function optimally. Dr. Chestnut did this by looking at what our ancestors ate before the prevalence of chronic illness arose in our society. He and other researchers have looked at the diet of olden day and modern day hunter-gatherers, who suffered from none of the chronic illnesses so prevalent today, to determine what we are genetically required to eat. As author and Ph.D. (Health) Loren Cordain writes, "[b]uilt into our genes is a blueprint for optimal nutrition—a plan that spells out the foods that make us healthy, lean, and fit."[71]

What are those foods? For starters, the answers to what constitutes a healthy diet are *not* found in recommended daily allowances (RDAs) or government-endorsed food guides. Nutrition expert and author Patrick Horford calls RDAs "the greatest lie in healthcare today."[72] Dr. Chestnut adds that "[c]urrent guidelines are based on required minimal amounts to avoid disease or maximal daily intakes based on toxicity levels, while eating the types of low fiber foods that were invalidly established as part of a healthy diet. The current guidelines have no healthy gold standard as a guide. The current guidelines use sickness and disease standards."[73] And Caldwell Esselstyn, M.D. explains in his book *Prevent and Reverse Heart Disease,* that, "There are powerful commercial interests that want no change in the American diet. Over the years, there have been a number of attempts to bring nutritional recommendations more into line with what the science actually shows. In every case, intensive lobbying by industry—the producers and purveyors of dairy products, meat, and poultry—has caused those who set the standards to pull their punches."[74]

Our ancestors ate what Dr. Chestnut calls the Innate Diet and what Dr. Cordain calls the Paleo Diet. These diets are rich in whole foods provided by nature, including vegetables, fruits, nuts, seeds, wild game and fish. Drs. Chestnut and Cordain assert that if you eat according to these diets, then you don't have to look at what particular food may help to reduce the risk of what particular disease. The right diet taken holistically will reduce the risk of all preventable diseases, and will increase your degree of health and vitality because it is loaded with nutrients that our genetic blueprint requires to express health.

Nowadays, however, the foods consumed by our ancestors have lower nutrient values and higher toxicity levels due to industrial agriculture and farming practices. Our air, water, and soil have been polluted by industrial living, and this affects the nutritional quality of our foods. Hence the importance of consuming organically grown and organically raised foods that are not laced with pesticides, herbicides, hormones, or other toxins. In some cases, even that won't be enough to achieve optimal nutrition, as will be explained in the section on supplementation below.

If you're eating the typical Western diet based on food groups and RDAs, with lots of processed foods, added sugar, and some fast food thrown in for good measure...well, you're not alone. That's the standard fare these days. But the good news is that you can change. You control what you put into your body, and you have an understanding of how important nutrition is to your quantity and quality of life and your effectiveness as a lawyer. So if you're ready to make a change and start eating a diet much closer to that of our ancestors, and much closer to what your cells genetically require, try these suggestions. Don't incorporate them all at once. Don't go from being a cheeseburger lover to a vegan overnight. That won't be sustainable. Ease into it, creating habits that will build on each other as you go.

Macronutrient Profile

Your diet consists of the macronutrients protein, carbohydrates, and fat. Set out below is the macronutrient profile of the typical Western or modern diet.

> ➤ Protein (industrially farmed,
>   fat-marbled meat and fish)   15-20%
> ➤ Carbohydrate (processed grains,
>   sugar, corn syrup)   45-55%
> ➤ Fat (grain fed meats, dairy, trans fats)   35-40%

To experience a higher degree of health and vitality in the biochemical dimension of life, slowly move toward the following macronutrient profile, which Dr. Chestnut calls the Innate Diet.

> ➤ Protein (vegetables and lean wild game)   20-35%
> ➤ Carbohydrate (fruits and vegetables)   25-40%
> ➤ Fat (organic meats and fish; vegetables, nuts) 30-45%[75]

Nutritional Supplements[76]

Even if you eat the perfect diet, due to modern living and agricultural practices, you're still likely to be deficient of three essential nutrients: Omega-3 fatty acids, probiotics, and vitamin D.

> ➤ *Omega-3 fatty acids*: These are required for the proper function of every cell, tissue, organ, and gland in the brain

and body. Deficiencies in Omega-3 fatty acids have been linked to several illnesses, such as ADHD in children; cancer, stroke, heart disease, diabetes, obesity, high blood pressure, depression, skin disorders, and digestive disorders in teens and adults; and to arthritis, osteoporosis, and Alzheimer's in the elderly. The only safe way to consume adequate levels of Omega-3 fatty acids is by supplementing your diet daily with purified Omega-3 fish oil.

➢ *Probiotics*: Probiotic bacteria are an essential requirement for proper immune system function, digestive system function, and vitamin production. Deficiencies in probiotic bacteria have been linked to several illnesses and conditions, such as digestive disorders, immune deficiency, cancer, heart disease, systemic infections, and decreased health and vitality. It is estimated that due to modern food production practices, we now consume less than *one millionth* of the amount of healthy probiotic bacteria required to maintain a healthy intestinal ecosystem. Dairy and agricultural sources of probiotics are insufficient to meet our genetically required needs; the only way to consume sufficient amounts of probiotic bacteria is through daily supplementation.

➢ *Vitamin D*: Modern industrial human beings are dangerously deficient in vitamin D. Deficiencies in vitamin D have been linked to diabetes, autism, asthma, and decreased immune function in infants and children; cancer, heart disease, MS, chronic bone and muscle pain, chronic inflammation, and decreased immune function in teens and adults; and osteoporosis, cancer, heart disease, and decreased immune function in the elderly. Since vitamin D is made in the skin from exposure to sunlight, unless you are getting 30 minutes of summer sunlight exposure over large parts of your body every day, you will most likely be deficient in vitamin D unless you supplement daily.

Deficiencies in any other vitamin, mineral, or nutrient for which you may be recommended to supplement are caused by dietary insufficiency. Seek to correct the deficiency through dietary sources rather than supplementing whenever possible.

Water

Drinking enough water is essential for good health. Our bodies are two-thirds water. We can die without water after just a few days (remember the lawyer in the desert from Chapter 3?). Thankfully, access to water is not an issue for most of us—but drinking enough of it certainly is. As a society we're chronically dehydrated. We drink lots of liquids—coffee, tea, milk, juice, pop, energy drinks, alcohol—but not a lot of water. There's a huge difference between liquids and water—all liquids are certainly *not* created equal.

Dehydration—even of the mild variety—can lead to constipation, headaches, lethargy, and mental confusion. These things aren't great for anybody—but it's especially hard to practice law effectively when you're confused and tired, suffering from a pounding headache, and dealing with stomach cramps! And those are just a *few* of the symptoms you may experience from not drinking enough water.

How much is enough? Most experts agree that the average person requires six to eight tall glasses of water a day—more if you're exercising vigorously. One way to determine the amount of water that's right for you is to drink half of your bodyweight—in ounces, not pounds, thankfully—daily. So if you weigh 150 pounds then drink 75 ounces of water each day.

Another great reason to drink water is that you'll eat less when you're well hydrated. We often mistake thirst for hunger. So a good strategy for hydration and for eating less is to drink one or two tall glasses of water before every meal or snack.

A great side effect of getting into the habit of drinking lots of water is that you'll get up from your desk more often—either to fill up your water bottle or to go pee! This movement will relieve your spine from long, continuous periods of sitting.

Lastly, make sure you're drinking the right kind of water. Tap water in many urban areas is not great at best and can be harmful at worst, so stick with natural mineral water, distilled water, filtered tap water, or bottled water.

Foods and toxins to decrease or eliminate

Eliminating or reducing your intake of these foods and toxins will go a long way to helping you experience enhanced health and vitality in the biochemical dimension of life.

> ➢ *Smoking*: I do not smoke and I never have, so I can only imagine how difficult it must be to quit. If you're a smoker and you don't value your health, that's one thing. But if you're a smoker and you want to live a long and healthy life, then you must quit smoking in order to be in integrity with that value. You might say that it's not as simple as that—but it is.
> ➢ *Fast food*: If you're like me, you've eaten your share of greasy, fried fast food (McDonalds, KFC, etc.) in your life. There's not much we can do about that now. But that doesn't mean you have to continue to eat it in the future. After all, while it may be fast, given all of the additives contained in it, is it really *food* at all? I encourage you to release fast food from your life once and for all. Eliminate it completely from the list of options you consider when dining out. Not 99% of the time (hard), but 100% of the time (easy). There are enough temptations in life that sap our attention and energy from time to time—don't let drive-thru hamburgers, fries, and popcorn chicken be among them.
> ➢ *Sugar*. Most lawyers will know that a diet high in sugar is a leading cause of obesity and diabetes. What you may not know, however, is that a diet high in sugar has also been found to reduce intelligence. Since intelligence is a key asset for any lawyer, keeping sugar in your diet to a minimum is just a smart thing to do. Sugar has also been linked to aggressive behavior, anxiety, ADHD, depression, eating disorders, and fatigue, among other ailments.[77] So as much as you can, get your sugar fix from fruit and stay away from foods containing added sugar (that includes most fruit juices) and its evil stepsisters: artificial sweeteners and high fructose corn syrup.

➢ *Stimulants (alcohol and caffeine)*: Like sugar (a stimulant in its own right), alcohol and caffeine also have been found to reduce intelligence. While many lawyers swear not only by their morning coffee, but also by their several other coffees throughout the day, caffeine diminishes concentration and memory. Since remembering things and concentrating on them are kind of important when preparing for trial or negotiating the finer points of a purchase agreement, consider cutting back on your trips to the coffee counter. Drink more water instead.

➢ *Dairy and Gluten*. You'll likely have noticed more dairy- and gluten-free labels on many packaged goods and on restaurant menus in the last couple of years. The reason is that many people are discovering that they are allergic or sensitive to these foods. Symptoms include sinus, digestive, and bowel issues. If you experience any of these issues on a sustained basis, consider a dairy-free and/or gluten-free diet for a month. The best case is that your issues clear up; the worst case is that you'll notice that most baked goods will be off-limits for the month, so you'll be forced to eat healthier alternatives most of the time. Even if your symptoms don't resolve, you might enjoy the smaller waistline that will likely result from a gluten- and/or dairy-free diet.

➢ *Drugs*. I will refrain from commenting on illegal drugs, other than to say that if you are a frequent user of them, you may likely require help beyond what this book can provide. As to legal, or pharmaceutical drugs, if you're on one or more renewable prescriptions for a chronic illness, consider what lifestyle choices you can make to remove the *cause* of that illness. Symptom-fighting drugs may be appropriate for the short term to give you time to make the changes to your cellular environment (through lifestyle choices like diet and exercise) necessary to allow your genes to express themselves differently. Remember, just because a drug may remove your symptoms, you are not necessarily healthier. It just means that you may be symptom-free; and if you do nothing to change your cellular environment while taking prescription drugs, sooner or later your body will send you another, even stronger signal (symptom) to get you to take notice. Under the allopathic paradigm, this may lead to more drug prescriptions, and the slippery slope is well underway. You'll then be involved in a never-ending game of Whack-a-Mole, trying to smack each symptom with a different drug every time it pops up.

If you find yourself playing that game, or in the line-up for it, know this: Studies have shown—including some published in the *Journal of the American Medical Association*—that between 120,000 and 300,000 people die in the Unites States every year from adverse reactions to prescription drugs.[78] In most cases, these are not people who took the wrong drugs or the wrong dose. These are people who took the right medicine, in the right dose, at the right time, as prescribed by their doctor. One study showed that 75 percent of these deaths were due to the inherent toxicity of the drugs rather than to allergic reactions.[79]

I am *not* recommending that you immediately cease taking prescription medicine prescribed by your medical doctor. I am, however, recommending that you seriously consider what you can do to remove the need to ingest toxic medications for the rest of your life by removing the cause of the symptoms for which the medicine has been prescribed. Start with lifestyle changes. It worked for Dean Ornish's atherosclerosis patients, and there's a good chance that it will work for you, too.

PSYCHOLOGICAL WELLNESS

The psychological dimension of life is how you think and what you think about. It's how you use your mind. Do you have clarity of thinking most of the time, or are you so stressed and overwhelmed that you find it hard to think straight? Do you have the confidence to handle the challenges that your career and every other social dimension of life will throw at you, or do you see every challenge as a gut-wrenching and stress-inducing test of your will and abilities? Do you have a positive self-image and high self-esteem, or are you constantly critical of yourself and unsure of your ability to function in today's fast-paced world? These are just some of the questions whose answers will inform your degree of psychological wellness.

For many, the psychological dimension is the trickiest of the three physiological dimensions of life. While exercising regularly and eating right may not be easy, those behaviors are at least easier to wrap your mind around than it is to figure out how to get your mind working optimally. Plus, the effects of diet and exercise are usually apparent to the eye, since they impact your appearance and the shape of your body. Therefore, your results in the physical and biochemical dimensions may be more tangible than in the psychological dimension.

Yet it's the psychological dimension of life that will probably have the biggest impact on your degree of health and vitality. Yes, the physical and biochemical dimensions are essential and important, but if you have to pick a starting point, it would be the psychological dimension. This is because the choice of what you do with your body and what you put into your body is made in your mind. It begins with the thought, *I will exercise* or *I will not exercise. I will eat this* or *I will not eat this.* Success in the physical and biochemical dimensions will greatly enhance your degree of success in the psychological dimension, because your brain works better when given essential nutrients and exercise. But where most lawyers experience the greatest amount of negative stress is in the psychological dimension of their lives. Therefore, success in the psychological dimension is the foundation of health and vitality in your life.

In my experience, a major source of negative psychological stress comes from a sense of being overwhelmed by the volume of our personal and professional responsibilities. It comes from expending undue energy on every daily decision, because you're just not sure what to do most of the time; you have no idea which decisions are good for you and which aren't—to the extent that you are conscious about your decisions at all. It comes from feeling like you're putting out fires every day rather than feeling like you're building or creating something meaningful every day. It comes from knowing that your time on this planet is ticking away, and because you're struggling to meet your daily obligations, you have no time to create a lasting legacy. It comes from feeling like you're navigating through life's journey with no compass, no roadmap, and no GPS of any kind. It comes from a sense of having little or no control over your life.

Holistic life plan

Much of this negative psychological stress can be eliminated with one simple strategy: creating a holistic life plan. It sounds so simple, but so few people invest the time and insight to actually do this. Many lawyers have a plan for their practice, and most law firms have a strategic plan for their firm, but almost no one takes the time—or even has the inclination—to develop a strategic plan for their *life*. When you think about it, what sense does that make? Isn't the purpose of a career to enhance, rather than erode, the quality of your life? Shouldn't we spend some serious time and energy mapping out what we want our *lives* to look like—our health, our career, our love relationship, our parenting, our finances, and so on—so we can work towards creating that ideal life?

And isn't this especially true for you, now that you know that all dimensions of life are interconnected and that you can't affect a part without affecting the whole? As discussed in Chapter 3, can you know how a choice or action will impact the degree of health and vitality in your life if you don't know how it will impact each different dimension of it? Now that you know what all of the dimensions of your life are (or you will know after creating your corporate wellness chart), you're in a position to create a plan for each dimension that fits within an overall life plan. While a life plan will give you many benefits, probably the most immediate and profound benefit you'll experience after creating your life plan is that you'll have given yourself the gift of a decision-making framework.

As you know, practicing law can and will suck up almost all of your time if you let it. That's because most lawyers don't have any sense of how their career is supposed to fit into their overall life. Most lawyers let their career be the tail that wags the dog that is their life! But when you have done some deep thinking and have developed a written strategic plan for every important category of your life, you start to see how your actions and choices in one category (your career, for example) affect other categories (like your level of health and fitness or your marriage). This also works the other way around: You gain a deep understanding of how your choices and actions relating to your health and fitness or your marriage affect your career. In short, you give yourself a context and a framework to make choices and decisions that make sense for your overall life, not just one aspect of it.

This is *so* important for lawyers when it comes to setting appropriate parameters or boundaries around their career (and around each dimension of life). What constitutes "appropriate" boundaries will differ for everyone depending on what their ideal life looks like. As you know, those boundaries will get tested every single day—that's the nature of practicing law; that's the nature of life. But arming yourself with a decision-making framework will give you the conviction to uphold those boundaries—to say yes only to the things that are congruent with your life plan, and no to all the things that are not. Most lawyers have never taken the time to sit down and think logically about why they are leading the life they are leading, and consequently, they have never created a holistic, strategic life plan. They haven't given themselves the precious, stress-melting gift of a decision-making framework. They haven't the slightest clue what boundaries need to be placed on their career to ensure that it enhances, rather than erodes, their overall quality of life. They let the tail wag the dog and they, unfortunately, experience the effects of that: high stress, health issues, unhappiness, lack of fulfillment, and decreased effectiveness as a lawyer.

I hear you. You're saying, *this is all great in theory, but how do I put this into practice?* Creating your "corporate" wellness chart is a great start. It will help you figure out all of the social dimensions of your life. You can also use it to assess the current level of integrity that you're bringing to your life by asking yourself, *am I investing the time, energy, and resources required to achieve a high level of wellness in each of these important dimensions of my life?* It is a hugely empowering and insightful exercise for you to complete, and it will set you up for immediate progress going forward in terms of your overall quality of life.

If you are really serious about creating a compelling, holistic life plan that covers all of the important dimensions of your life— your health, career, family, finances, social life, etc.—you need to get away from the demands of your daily life for a few days and give yourself the space to really go deep and examine what you want your life to look like and what you want to achieve during your short time on this planet. You need to figure out not only what you want, but also why you want it—the purpose behind your desires—and whether or not you're willing to pay the price to get it. Before you can do any of that, you need to figure out what your foundational beliefs are in each category of your life, because your beliefs will dictate the actions you need to take to achieve the life you want. And, importantly, you'll need to record your life plan in a manner that is instructional, adaptable, and emotional. As one lawyer and author has put it, "[w]ithout forming a road map for his career and life, a lawyer is just floundering around and reacting to chance events."[80]

The best—if not the only—system in the world to help you do this is called Lifebook.

While it's a whole lot more than this, essentially Lifebook is a four-day strategic life planning retreat that guides you to discover and document your premise, vision, purpose, and strategy in 12 important categories of your life. By the end of the four days, you will have created your own lifebook: the blueprint for what your ideal life looks like and your action plan for creating it.

Lifebook is innovative, logical, and practical—just the way that all good lawyers think. It recognizes that every extraordinary achievement in the history of humankind was created using the following four-step process:

1. Identify and clarify your vision (what you want to achieve)
2. Create your plan to achieve it
3. Take action to achieve it
4. Measure and report your progress, and adjust if necessary

The people who built the pyramids, who put a man on the moon, and who created the iPad all used this process. Your law firm probably uses this process as part of its strategic planning, too.

But have you ever used it for your practice? Do you know, precisely and with clarity, what you want your practice to look like in five or 10 years? How much will you be working, how much will you be billing, what clients or kinds of clients will you be working with, how much money will you be making, how much time off will you take, what changes in the legal services landscape will require changes in your practice? And have you deeply thought through how all of this will impact the rest of your life?

What if you were to do this deep thinking across all important categories or social dimensions of your life? Can you imagine the clarity and control you would gain over your life? And could you imagine all of the stress that would melt away as a result?

You won't have to imagine it, because you can—and must—measure it. Lifebook allows you to do this by taking and re-taking their proprietary holistic lifestyle assessment that measures over 120 indicators of wellness and quality of life. It quantifies something that is very difficult to quantify: your level of wellness in every dimension of life, including the psychological dimension. This helps you measure your progress and adjust your course, if necessary, from time to time.

There is now a lawyers-only stream of the Lifebook system, called Lifebook for Lawyers. You can learn more about it, and you can access the Lifebook lifestyle assessment, at www.wellnesslawyer.com.

There are of course other best practices for wellness in the psychological dimension of life besides creating a holistic life plan, some of which may form part of the strategies you choose for improving your mindset in the course of creating your life plan.

Meditation

Meditation is one such best practice. If you meditate regularly already, that's wonderful—keep it up. But if you're anything like I was until recently, you've heard about meditation and have spoken to people who swear by it, but you just don't get it. *Sitting around for a half hour cross-legged and chanting or breathing funny...how is that supposed to help me? That's for Buddhist monks and yogis; it's not for me.* I don't blame you. For years I said it wasn't for me, either. But that was because I didn't fully appreciate the benefits of practicing meditation. Isn't that really why we do anything in life? We do things because the benefits of doing them outweigh the benefits of not doing them. When you understand the benefits of meditation, and you're serious about your desire to achieve a high degree of health and vitality, then it becomes hard *not* to meditate regularly.

Before the benefits, however, let's dispel the myths. Meditation is not a religion; it's not cultish, and it doesn't need to involve chanting, deep breathing, sitting cross-legged, listening to strange music, or wearing funny clothes. All it requires is silence and stillness and a few minutes of your time. It needn't take up an hour or even a half hour of your day. As with exercise, 10 minutes, 20 minutes, or even just a few minutes a day is better than nothing. All you need to do is find a quiet place and focus on your breathing to help clear your mind of the endless clutter that finds its way in there every day. Of course, you won't clear it completely, especially the first few times (or even the first few dozen times) you meditate, but if you make it a habit, over time you'll get better and better at it. Your mind will become stronger and stronger. In this sense, your mind is just like any muscle in your body: If you exercise it regularly it will gain strength and function better.

The authors of *The Happy Lawyer* write of meditation this way: "If you are inclined to dismiss mindfulness meditation as some sort of New Age mumbo jumbo, you will have to ignore a number of studies that show meditation programs of eight-weeks or less reduce anxiety and depression, while increasing well-being and immune system responses."[81]

Philosopher and entrepreneur (and law school drop-out) Brian Johnson is an avid student and practitioner of meditation. According to his research and personal experience, he identified these as the top five benefits of meditation:

1. It strengthens your mind, and allows you to put your mind *where* you want, *when* you want (a skill that positive

psychologists have identified as essential to enhancing happiness).

2. It helps you build will power and self-discipline by strengthening your pre-frontal cortex.
3. It boosts your immune system by inducing the relaxation response (for example, it helps get you out of the "fight or flight" response in which most of us spend our days).
4. It causes your genes to express themselves in a healthier way.
5. It helps you connect to the highest version of yourself.[82]

Does anyone *not* want more of that good stuff in their life?

If you want to achieve optimal health, meditation really isn't an option—it's an essential ingredient. And if the term meditation scares you off, as was formerly the case with me[83], then just call it "still time" or "breathing exercises." The point is not what it's called; the point is the benefits that you'll reap from practicing meditation regularly.

If you're a chronic multi-tasker and you just can't get your head around the idea of sitting still and focusing on your breathing for 15 minutes, then consider a yoga class, which often combines deep breathing and meditation with core and strength training. Eat a salad after class and you'll have scored a hat trick of positive physical, biochemical, and psychological stress in an hour. How can that *not* make you a more effective lawyer for the rest of the day?

Daily Affirmations

Another best practice in the psychological dimension is to create a daily affirmation or intention and read it every morning, preferably out loud. A good affirmation or intention will involve a connection to your purpose and will remind you of the kind of day you want to experience. It will get you in a positive, purposeful mindset for the day, which will help you achieve your goals and overcome any obstacles that get in your way. It will help you stay focused on what's most important, and to resist all of the people and things that will try to sidetrack you on a daily basis. Plus, it will just make you feel good, plain and simple.

In the Best of the Blog section of the book, there is an article about affirmations that includes a portion of my daily affirmation. That might help you craft your own if you've never done so before. It's called "Affirmations can make you a hero."

Another article that I've included in the Best of the Blog section of the book, entitled "How do you slow...down...time?" is about how, when you get really conscious about how you live your life (by creating a strategic, holistic life plan and by living in integrity with it), you find that time actually slows down. Your life doesn't fly by in an instant; you find more appreciation for daily life, and you are able to take in so much more of what life has to offer. All of this enhances your degree of health and vitality in the psychological dimension of life.

Other best practices

There are many other best practices in the psychological dimension of life. Since the majority of life's social dimensions will relate to your mindset, thinking, and the amount of stress you may experience in the psychological dimension, let's move on to discuss some best practices in the key social dimensions of life.

7

BEST PRACTICES IN THE
SOCIAL DIMENSIONS OF LIFE

You will recall from Chapter 4 that the social dimensions of life are the different aspects or categories of your life that impact your ability to function in society at your highest level and to live your best life. While the physiological dimensions of life apply to everyone, the social dimensions will be different for each lawyer.

In this chapter, I will discuss some best practices in the social dimensions that will appear in the lives of *most* lawyers. Before you read this chapter, however, I encourage you to re-read the lead-in to Chapter 6, as it contains important contextual information that applies to this chapter as well.

PHYSICAL WELLNESS

In the social dimension context, physical wellness usually relates to fitness and diet. Each of these has been discussed in the section on physiological best practices, but here I'll add one more benefit you'll experience as an effect of exercising regularly and eating well, in terms of making you a more effective lawyer: You'll gain enhanced confidence.

Exercise and proper nutrition make you look and feel better. They improve your self-esteem. They require a high degree of self-discipline, commitment, and resolve that will translate into your work habits as well. All of these effects of a good diet and regular physical activity will give you more confidence in the practice of law. As Calgary lawyer Diana Richmond says, "If you look good and feel good, you will have more confidence and this will create a positive environment in your workplace."

Let's face it, appearance is important in the practice of law. And appearance is not just the way you dress—it's the way your body looks underneath those clothes. Jonathan Mraunac, an associate at Foran Glennon Palandech Ponzi & Rudloff in Chicago and Chair of the Health & Wellness Committee of the Young Lawyers Section of the Chicago Bar Association, explains: "In law, appearance is big, and when you take care of yourself, you look better. A healthy appearance creates a positive feedback loop. Lawyers are expected to always be on the ball, to be story tellers and entertainers, to dress impeccably...when you're physically fit it's not as much of a burden to get up for this everyday. If you don't have good habits, it becomes harder."

In many areas of law, lawyers will look to exploit any weakness in the other side's case, position, or argument. While it may not be politically correct to say, the truth is that being overweight and out of shape can be construed as a weakness. Practicing law is difficult enough. Do you need the added difficulty of reduced confidence due to a weight problem or poor body shape that's caused by sedentary living and a poor diet? Matthew Moriarty, a partner in Tucker Ellis' Cleveland office makes the point this way: "I wake up every day with 50 problems, but being 30 pounds overweight and out of shape isn't one of them."

When you have a physically strong and lean physical appearance—and the mental fortitude and self-confidence that goes along with that—you're likely to be the lawyer your clients and colleagues will turn to for key projects. In that sense, it not only makes you a more effective lawyer, it gives you the *opportunity* to be a more effective lawyer. If you want more business, being in great shape will help you get it. And perhaps more importantly, when you have the self-confidence and strength of mind that results from a high level of physical wellness, when you say no to business or no to partners wanting to assign you work because your professional plate is already full, they won't question you. This gives you a much higher ability to set boundaries around your work life and to uphold those boundaries with conviction. The result is that you'll gain more time to devote to your physical health and vitality.

Having this high level of self-confidence creates a positive, healthy feedback loop that spans all dimensions of your life, not just your career. As Mraunac says, "It lessens social anxiety. And when you're single, you have to take care of yourself to attract the opposite sex." Which is a nice segue into the social dimension we'll look at next: family wellness.

FAMILY WELLNESS

The family dimension of life will include your relationship with your spouse, your kids, your own parents and siblings, and to a lesser extent, your extended family. Some lawyers may wish to separate each of these into a separate social dimension on which to focus. For instance, you may wish to make your love relationship and your parenting separate dimensions because each is of such vital importance to your quality of life.

If you have a spouse or children, you know that some of life's greatest joys and stresses occur in the family dimension of life. If your love relationship isn't working right, then nothing in your life seems to work right. If any of your kids experience significant health, drug use, or other behavioral issues, nothing else seems to matter. And on the flip side, when your marriage is humming along beautifully and you're spending time laughing and playing with your kids, nothing else seems to matter either.

Hopefully you experience personal enjoyment and fulfillment from your law practice, but for most of us, the main reason we practice law is to provide for our family and to help create a higher quality of life for them. But, as you know, lawyering can get so all-consuming at times that you often spend far less meaningful time with your spouse and kids than you want to and than *they* want you to. And when that happens—especially if that becomes the rule rather than the exception—it becomes a huge stressor in your life that adversely affects your health and your effectiveness as a lawyer.

As the authors of *The Happy Lawyer* concluded after their in-depth study of the art and science of happiness generally, and as it relates to lawyers, "the best path to happiness lies *in the direction of family and community*."[84]

Build family into your life plan

A great marriage or raising great kids isn't a game of chance; these things don't just happen. You need a plan for them. You have to invest focused time and energy to develop, maintain, grow, and evolve your relationship with your spouse and kids. You're always changing, your spouse is always changing, and more than anyone, your kids are always changing. So not only do you need a plan for a great marriage and a great family, you need to monitor and adapt your plan often—probably more often than your planning for any other social dimension of your life. Keep that in mind when you create and implement your strategic life plan. Knowing how your choices and actions in every other dimension of your life affect the quality of your love relationship and parenting (and your relationships with your own parents and siblings, too) is imperative to achieving success in the family dimension. For instance, understanding how a high level of physical fitness can make you a better lover and a better parent will impact not only your physical dimension of life, but your family dimension, too. Same goes for your career. When you have cultivated a passionate love relationship or have become an amazing mom or dad to your kids, that makes you want to spend more time with them and less time at the office. At the same time, you know that you have to take care of your work commitments and meet your billing targets (whether self- or firm-imposed) so that you can provide for your family. Having the keen, conscious sense of this balance that results from having a written and well-thought out holistic life plan makes you more focused and effective at work *and* at home.

Dr. David Jackson, father of three teenage daughters, says that he gets so much leverage in his life from understanding at a deep level what kind of father he wants to be to his kids. His desire to be a great role model and to leave a lasting legacy for his children drives everything else in his life. It makes him want to go to work as a chiropractor and entrepreneur every day to create value and improve the quality of people's lives, which in turn improves the quality of his family life. It makes him want to be in great shape, so that he minimizes the chances of dying early and missing out on the still-to-come great moments in his daughters' lives. It makes him want to have an epic love relationship with his wife, so that his daughters can see first hand what a proper loving marriage looks like. For Dr. Jackson, creating a life plan (he used the Lifebook system to do this) literally took his life from good to extraordinary, and all of the leverage he needed to do that came from the parenting section of his plan.

Weekly date nights with your spouse

Life as a lawyer is so hectic, and if you add kids to the mix, it's even crazier. Finding meaningful, one-on-one time to connect with your spouse can be difficult. It's easy for you and your spouse to become like two passing ships in the night if you don't make it a point to disconnect from the rest of the world and to connect with each other. The quality of your love relationship is foundational to your quality of life, so if you want a life of health, happiness, and fulfillment, your love relationship can't be left to chance. Just like your health, your law practice, or anything else in your life that matters, your love relationship requires consistent action to achieve success. Weekly date nights are one great way to do this. It's best to make it the same day every week, and to build your week around date night, rather than to scramble every week to fit a date into your busy schedule.

Committing to this sacred connection time with your lover every week will do more to keep your love relationship well than pretty much anything else you can do. The key is consistent action. Date night happens *every week*—no exceptions. You're not only going to love the dates, but also the profound, positive effect they have on your relationship and your overall happiness and quality of life. This week, spend a few minutes with your spouse to pick the day of the week that best fits your schedule for date night. Then commit to each other that nothing else will take priority over your date night. If you pick Wednesday night, for example, then no work, kid stuff, board meetings, in-law visits, nor anything else will get in the way of your Wednesday date night. Tell the people you need to tell that Wednesday is your date night, and it's off limits to anything *but* date night. And most importantly, plan your first date night. Get a sitter, make reservations, and pick out something nice to wear. Do something you haven't done in a while or go somewhere you haven't been in a while. Make it special, romantic, and passionate—make it so that both of you can't wait until *next* Wednesday night!

Parenting

I have three wonderful kids, and at the time of this writing, I have a fourth on the way. Parenting is the definition of paradox for me. It is such a mix of awesome and aargh! Of gratitude and grrrr! I practiced law for 12 years and I run several businesses, but parenting is the most important job I'll ever have. It's certainly the most rewarding—and the most demanding.

I thank my lucky stars every day for my kids. I know how privileged I am to watch them grow up every day. They provide life's most memorable moments. But, even with all that said, what a *challenge* it is to parent those kids! Sometimes they suck every last ounce of energy right out of me. Sometimes it seems as if it's a never-ending test of wills and patience. The resilience they have to test my boundaries on a daily—no, hourly—basis is truly mind-boggling. If I'm not on my game *all* the time, these little people know exactly how to knock me off it. And it's *such* a fine line between being on my game and being thrown completely off the rails. Those adorable, cuddly, beautiful little creatures…they sure can wear me down. That is, of course, until they bring me right back up again.

If you're a parent, I'm sure you can relate to all of this. You know how wonderful, difficult, rewarding, and challenging raising kids can be. You know that life's best moments usually involve your children. You want to be there for them not only now, but for many years to come. Yet, practicing law has an annoying habit of getting in the way of all of that. When work prevents you from spending the amount of time you want to spend with your kids, you not only don't get to experience the joys of being with your kids, you experience sadness, resentment, or anger at your job for preventing that. Those feelings create added stress, which makes you less focused and effective at work. Losing focus means it takes you longer to get your work done, and you don't create as much value for your clients. Then, the whole cycle starts again. I don't have any one-size-fits-all solutions here. But allow me to suggest a couple of things.

First, your life plan should bring to the surface the need to be a great role model for your kids. If you want to raise happy, healthy kids, you'll have a much better chance of success if *you* are happy and healthy. Second, your life plan should describe how much time you want to spend with your kids on a daily basis. Many moms and dads who work as lawyers feel guilty about not spending enough time with their kids. Where does that guilt come from? If it comes from not spending the amount of time that *you* want to spend with your kids, then the guilt could be warranted. But if it comes from some external view that you should spend a certain amount of time with your kids every day, then check your guilt at the door. Quality of time and attention with your kids is much more important than quantity. Time block quality time with your kids—even if it's only 15 minutes here or there. But make that time interruption-free. Separate focused work time from focused parenting time.

This is where boundaries come in—but boundaries work both ways. Make it clear to your kids the importance of work and the value that you bring to them by working, so that they know your time away from them is needed and is actually an expression of love for them, not the opposite. That way, it's easier to explain to your children why you can't always be home for dinner or at their soccer game or piano recital. But, at the same time, remember that it's those moments and memories—and not the details of an asset purchase agreement or mezzanine financing—that will matter when you consider the legacy of your life. As with most everything, the interplay between work time and kid time is about finding the right balance. A holistic life plan is an essential first step to achieving that balance.

So that's the big picture stuff on parenting. Here's one small, but profound, parenting strategy that I have implemented to take stock of how I've performed as a parent at the end of each day. I simply ask myself, "Was I a good Dad today?"

Some days the answer is an obvious yes. Some days it's a clear no. But most days, I need to give it some thought before I answer. I take a quick inventory of my interactions with each child that day, and I self-assess. Was I present with them? Was I loving? Encouraging? Teaching? Fun? Did I keep my cool? Did I help them keep theirs? Was I a good role model for them today?

If a daily habit to self-assess your parenting appeals to you, ask yourself every night before bed "Was I a good Mom or Dad today?" And—here's the key—never answer no two days in a row.

SOCIAL WELLNESS

"Next to sex, socializing is the activity that makes us happiest."[85] How's that for context?

While most lawyers appreciate the importance of health, career, family, and finances in their lives, few fully appreciate the importance of surrounding themselves with the right friends. The non-family members you spend your time with have a tremendous influence on the level of health and vitality in your life. In a study that looked at what sort of interactions make us happiest, interactions with friends scored highest, slightly above interactions with spouses and children, and well above interactions at work or time spent alone. Other research suggests that about 70 percent of our controllable happiness comes from relationships.[86]

Jim Rohn famously said that you are the average of the five people with whom you spend the most time. This applies to your health, your career, your finances, and so on. If you surround yourself with healthy people, you're more likely to be healthy. If you surround yourself with people who have achieved success in their career, you're more likely to find career success yourself. If you hang out with people who have achieved financial abundance, you're more likely to achieve it, too.

Plus, life is just more fun when you're around positive, upbeat, charismatic, fun people—and it's less fun when your surrounded by negative, complaining, downers most of the time.

You're going to have lifelong friends you've known since you were a kid. Some of these friendships will be enriching for life, and some will be less so. There's no need to break up with your less uplifting friends; but there's no need to go out of your way to spend more time with them, either. So if you take Jim Rohn's idea to heart, it's not about cutting loose the bottom feeders in your life as much as it is about seeking out mentors and other people who have achieved success in areas where you desire further growth. This certainly applies to your law practice. I was fortunate to have some wonderful role models amongst the senior lawyer ranks when I was a junior lawyer. When I first began to practice, I was assigned a principal mentor from whom I learned a great deal not only about the practice of law, but also about how to practice law within the context of a balanced wellness lifestyle. When you see it done with your own eyes, you're much more likely to believe it can be done and to create that in your own practice and life. If you're a junior lawyer and you don't have such a mentor or role model already, seek one out. Most senior lawyers are happy to impart wisdom to their younger colleagues, and they will appreciate the initiative you've shown to seek them out.

Of course, you're not going to enjoy spending time with all of the people in your firm, and you'll likely be forced to spend time with some people you don't enjoy from time to time. That's the nature of practice and it's the nature of life. But do your best to minimize interactions with people who bring you down, and if your workplace is full of those kinds of people, either look for another place to work, or make sure you have lots of uplifting, positive friends outside the office—and make it a point to spend time with them. As with your love relationship and your parenting, use time blocking to build positive social engagements into your schedule. Treat them with the same sanctity as client meetings; don't blow them off at the first sign of your desk piling up. Blow off your friends too many times and they won't be friends anymore.

Another best practice when considering your social wellness is to make a list of characteristics you want in your friends and, equally important, a list of things you won't tolerate. If humor, dependability, and responsiveness are the qualities you value in a friend, don't let anyone into your inner circle who doesn't have these traits. And if you can't tolerate people who complain all the time about things, but never do anything to change them, then learn to say "no thanks" when these people show up in your life and want to take some of your time. As a lawyer, you have less free time than most people; you can't afford to spend any of it with people who don't make a positive contribution to your life in some way. If you do, that's time away from your work, from your family, from your health and fitness, and from your other important commitments. It's just not worth it. You need to be vigilant about this. Being clear and certain about whom you share your time with and whom you don't makes you a more effective lawyer and a healthier, happier, and more fulfilled person.

FINANCIAL WELLNESS

The financial dimension of life is one area in which many lawyers have some sort of plan in place already. Money is important, both now and in the future, and most lawyers get that. I don't pretend to be a financial planning expert, and this book is not about financial planning, but I would like to share two best practices that may not have occurred to most lawyers (and most financial planners, for that matter). The first is getting clear on the *purpose* of money in your life. The second is the oft-forgotten idea that the real key to financial wellness isn't how much money you make—it's how much money you keep.

Purpose of money

Have you ever thought deeply about the purpose of money in your life? Yes, you need it to buy things, and you need it to provide the necessities of life for you and your loved ones—and hopefully a few things beyond the simple necessities, as well. But do you know exactly how much money you need? How much money you want? Both now and in the future? And, more importantly, do you know exactly *why* you want that amount of money—what you're going to use that money for?

We'd all love to have millions of dollars in the bank, right? But do you know how, exactly, having millions does or would make your life better? There are people with $10,000 in the bank that are healthier, happier, and more fulfilled than people with

$10,000,000. And there are people with $10,000,000 in the bank that are healthier, happier, and more fulfilled than people with $10,000. So money is not the determining factor when it comes to quantity and quality of life.

The key to figuring out the purpose of money in your life is an understanding that money has no inherent value. You can't eat money, you can't drink money, and—unless you're an architect who is a few tools short of a toolbox—you can't use bills and coins to build shelter. Money only has value when it is exchanged for something that improves your quality of life. So the real question about money is, how much of it do you need to provide the quality of life you desire? Having $10,000,000 sounds wonderful, and it might well be, but what price are you willing to pay to get it? If making millions comes at a sacrifice to the degree of health and vitality you experience in your life, is it worth it?

Tim Ferriss writes in *The 4-Hour Workweek* that the old school view of money, held by people he calls "deferrers," is to make a ton of it. But the new school view of money held by people Ferriss calls the "new rich" is to make a ton of it "with specific reasons and defined dreams to chase, timelines and steps included."[87] The key question, Ferriss writes, is what are you working *for*?

The prevailing business model of law practice won't allow you to work four-hour weeks, but don't get fooled by the title. Ferriss' views on the purpose of money are spot on no matter how many hours a week you work; in fact they're more relevant the *more* hours a week you work. Since time and attention are the real currencies of life, the more time and attention you spend acquiring money, the more expensive that money is to acquire. Who's richer, the person who makes $200,000 working 80-hour weeks, the person who makes $100,000 working 40-hour weeks, or the person who makes $50,000 working 20-hour weeks? The answer is whoever makes the money required to enjoy the quality of life they desire in the manner that least sacrifices the quality of life they desire.

Enter the holistic life plan again. A financial plan is worthless unless it fits within an overall life plan. A financial plan to acquire millions for retirement is useless if it costs your health and relationships to get it. But when you have thought through your finances deeply and know exactly what purpose money plays in your life and what you want to use your money for—with more clarity than you've ever brought to this exercise in the past—you'll be able to plan your career and investments around how much money you want. That will make you more focused and efficient on the job, and happier and more fulfilled in life.[88]

As Steven Harper writes about extensively in *The Lawyer Bubble*, a great many lawyers get caught up in a game of whoever makes the most money wins. Their competitive nature takes over and they lose sight of the cost of earning their enormous salaries. This is due in part to the public nature of salaries now. At many firms, all partners know how much every other partner is earning, and trade magazines publish compensation metrics such as average profits per partner for the biggest firms. Consequently, many lawyers mistakenly tie self-worth to net worth, even though these are two very separate and distinct things. There is no winning the whoever makes the most money wins game: There will always be another lawyer who makes more money than you.

But when you have a financial plan within an overall life plan, the rules of the game shift from whoever makes the most money wins, to *this is what my ideal life looks like, this is how much money that will require, and this is the amount of time and attention I'm prepared to invest to earn it.* Upon creating a life plan in this manner, some lawyers will realize that growing their practice is required, others will realize that they need to scale back, and still others may have to simply tweak what they already have going.

The parable about the Mexican fisherman and American businessman is the best illustration I have ever come across about the importance of knowing the purpose of money in your life. The full parable is included in *The 4-Hour Workweek* and I recommend you read it. It's about a Mexican fisherman who sleeps late, fishes a little, plays with his children, takes a siesta with his wife, and strolls into the village every evening, where he sips wine and plays guitar with his amigos; and it's about the American businessman who tells the fisherman that he could help him grow his fishing business over the next 25 years and make millions of dollars, so that when the fisherman retires he could sleep late, fish a little, play with his children, take a siesta with his wife, and stroll into the village every evening to sip wine and play guitar with his amigos.[89]

The point is, don't assume that more is better. Get clear on how much the things you want cost. Don't earn it and then ask, *what am I going to do with it?* When you do that, you'll end up spending your money on meaningless stuff and ask *where did all the money go?* Figure out what you want to do with money, then earn it. This will make you more focused and effective—and you might find that you won't have to work as long and as hard as you thought in order to achieve what you want. You'll end up with the quality of life you want with a lot less stress.

Keeping more money

Earning money is only one half of the equation—the less important half. The more important question is how much you keep. One of the reasons that many lawyers keep sacrificing so much—long hours, eroding health, little time for friends and family—is that they have created a lifestyle that consumes all of the money they earn every year—sometimes even more. They may earn hundreds of thousands or even millions of dollars a year, but it all goes out the door as quickly—or more quickly—than it comes in.

I have seen this happen in my life (not the making millions part, but the spending more than I made part). When I articled (the apprenticeship year for lawyers in Canada between law school and admission to practice) in 1999-2000 I made $28,000. Over my next dozen years in practice my salary multiplied many times over, but I often think that I never had so much money as when I articled. My expenses were low: no kids, no mortgage, no loans (law school in Canada is much cheaper than in the United States—especially back then). Over the years, I got married, started a family, got a mortgage, bought a couple of cars, started a college fund for the kids, put a bunch of insurance in place, went on some trips … you get the picture. I spent money to the point that the more I made every year, the less I had. Expenses exceeded income for a few years. I learned that credit lines are a wonderful and dangerous thing.

I know I'm not alone in this. And while I never made a million dollars or more a year practicing law, some lawyers who do are in the same boat. The reason for this is Parkinson's Law, which states that unless active steps are put in place to prevent it, your expenses will always rise to meet your income. Always—no matter how much money you make. And when this happens, you experience the opposite of financial freedom: You are trapped by your lifestyle into continuing to chase more money, no matter the cost or personal sacrifice of doing so—just so you can stay afloat. This can happen to millionaires and billionaires just as it can with "thousandaires." It causes a massive erosion of health, vitality, and quality of life.

It would make sense to me if a lawyer consciously decided that she would work her butt off—80, 100, 120 hour weeks—from age 25 to 35 making an average of, say, $200,000 per year after taxes during that time—while keeping expenses down to $50,000 per year. At the end of those 10 years, the lawyer would have $1,500,000 in the bank, assuming she had no investment loss or growth, and she could write her own ticket from there. She could transition to lower-paying part-time work and then have time to enjoy the fruits of her labors of the past 10 years for the rest of her life. There would be some negative health, vitality, and quality of life issues during those 10 years, but they could probably be made up for over the course of the next 40-plus years of her life.

Do you know any lawyer who has done this? Or do most of the lawyers you know live at the mercy of Parkinson's Law with no financial or occupational freedom—and the increased negative stress that brings—because their next draw or paycheck will be quickly spent, if it hasn't been spent already.

The thing is, most of the expenses we incur don't actually improve our quality of life in any tangible way. When you haven't consciously thought about the purpose of the things and experiences you want, as well as the cost of those things and experiences, you end up spending money on things and experiences just because other people do. So here, again, the life plan is essential.

The truth is, in order to get out from under Parkinson's Law, you need a budget and you need to stick to that budget—no matter how much money you make. As business-building guru Brian Tracy advises his students, you need to drive a *wedge* between your income and expenses. For the golfers among you, I would suggest keeping a wedge in your office so that you see it every day to remind you of this most important law of financial freedom. Once you have created your budget, take five minutes each day to track your spending, and have 15-minute weekly financial reviews with your spouse, so that you both know where you stand. You spend so much of your time earning money; doesn't it make sense to spend a few extra minutes to make sure you keep more of it?

Invest in your wellness

I'd like to cover one more point in this section before moving on. It may not actually belong in this section about the financial dimension of life, but I've put it here anyway because it's about investing. It's not about investing in stocks, or bonds, or real estate, however. It's about investing in your wellness.

It's critical to understand that the time, energy, and resources you allocate to your degree of health and vitality are not spent—they are invested. Investment is the right word here because the time, energy, and resources you invest will generate tremendous return on investment for you and your loved ones. You have probably heard the phrase before that you are your most important asset. This is particularly true for lawyers who generally only get paid when they show up for work—and it's pretty hard to work (and impossible to work effectively) when you're not healthy. Investing in yourself gives you increased earning power by increasing your effectiveness now and by increasing your ability to continue to be effective throughout the future.

Think of it this way. You probably have investments in a 401(k) or RRSP that you have earmarked for later use, when you turn 65 or whatever age you decide to stop working full-time. You have taken money that you could have spent today and put it aside for your use at a later time. Most every financial planner on the planet will tell you this is the right thing to do—and it very well may be. But what if by the time you get to be 65 your health is in such a bad state that you can't enjoy that money you worked so hard for and sacrificed so much for during all those years? What if you can't take all those trips you'd been planning due to preventable health issues (and remember, the vast majority of health issues *are* preventable)? Or what if you're not around at 65 at all? What good are your financial investments to you then?

Your clients don't hold a mortgage on your life. As a recently retired lawyer friend of mine often says, how many clients will show up at your funeral?

CAREER WELLNESS

This book has made the point several times that there are many other equally (if not more) important dimensions of your life than your career. But that does not mean your career is not extremely important to your overall wellness and quality of life. There are many reasons for this, but the primary one is that during your time as a practicing lawyer, you'll spend more time on your career than anything else in your life. While we know that most lawyers work more—many a lot more—than this, let's assume that lawyers average an 8-hour workday. So one third of every day (putting aside weekends and holidays for the moment) is allocated to your career. Another third or close to it is (or should be) spent sleeping. That means that most lawyers spend 50 percent of the time that they are awake working. Of course, many lawyers spend a lot more than that. I once had a colleague who *billed* over 4,000 hours in one year—that's almost half of the total hours in an entire year! If you're not spending that time in a way that makes you happy and fulfilled, or that enhances your health and vitality, it's difficult to have a high quality of life.

Love it, hate it, or just okay?

There are plenty of lawyers who cannot stand practicing law. They hate it every day they practice, all day long. If you're one of those lawyers, and you have given the practice a chance to grow on you (for example, you've practiced for at least a couple of years and you've tried different aspects of practice), you need to find another career—and fast. There are lots of books and experts who can help you do that. If you absolutely loathe the practice of law, then we can't even begin to have a conversation about career wellness, other than to say that you don't have any. Or more correctly, you have a very low degree of it.

But this book is not aimed at those lawyers. The purpose of this book is not to convince all lawyers to quit their jobs and find other careers. As mentioned at the outset, lawyers are essential to the orderly functioning of society. Without lawyers, chaos and anarchy would ensue. So we can't all quit—nor should we.

There are lawyers reading this book who absolutely love practicing law. If you're one of those lawyers, to you I say congratulations. There are very few people on this planet who love what they do for a living, and if you're one of them, you're lucky—no, deserving. I hope that this book has and will help you to increase your level of wellness in other dimensions of your life, and to achieve an enhanced overall quality of life.

I suspect, however, that most lawyers reading this book *like* practicing law; they don't have a sense of malaise every morning when the wake up and head to work, but they don't do cartwheels on the way there, either. Some days are great, some are terrible, and most are good, or maybe just okay. If you're one of those lawyers (I was when I practiced full-time) then you may be what Tim Ferriss describes as dying a "slow spiritual death over 30-40 years of tolerating the mediocre."[90] If you lack passion for the practice, you might be better off quitting and turning your real passions into a business opportunity. I can't tell you whether that's for you or not. But what I can suggest is that quitting is not the only option. If you're a lawyer who describes your career as "okay," and you still want to practice law for the foreseeable future, then you need to do one of two things to achieve a higher level of career wellness.

The first is to find a way to learn to love practicing law. If for you lawyering is just okay, then there are things you like about it and things you don't. Figure out what you like and what you don't, and do more of the things you like and less of the things you don't. Pick the area or issue that most intrigues you, and become an expert at it. If the practice of law is what you like, but you don't like the pressures and politics of big firm life, go to a smaller firm. If recording your time is the bane of your existence, then look for an in-house position. Whatever you do, don't complain about certain aspects of the practice, but then never do anything about them. Truly intelligent lawyers do not put up with perpetual pain in their lives; when they identify a recurring source of pain in their career (or in the rest of their lives) that develops into suffering, they do something about it. Pain is unavoidable; suffering is not.

The second way for you to achieve a higher level of career wellness is to learn to love what the practice of law brings to your life. In other words, if you don't love the ins and outs of the practice, you need to be crystal clear on the exact ways that lawyering improves your overall quality of life. You need to consciously identify the purpose of your career, and draw a clear and unequivocally positive link from your career to your quality of life. When you know exactly the purpose that practicing law plays in your life—whether that's to earn a good income to provide for your family, for the intellectual challenge, to help your clients achieve a desired result, or to make the world a better place—it makes you more focused and effective.

It's amazing how many lawyers have never systematically thought through that question. Knowing with clarity the purpose that your career plays in your life is *so* important, because when you're doing the stuff that you don't love—and let's admit, there's plenty of mind-numbing aspects of practicing law—your *purpose* gives you the intestinal fortitude to get through it. When you know there are other aspects of the practice that you *do* love and you know that the benefits of your job far outweigh the drawbacks, it makes it much easier to accept the lesser parts of the job when you can't change them. Without purpose, we tend to dwell on the bad stuff. But when we're not distracted by the bad stuff—by complaining and wishing things were not so—we become more effective lawyers.

Creating your holistic life plan is, of course, essential to clearly defining the purpose of your career, since your purpose will probably relate to other dimensions of your life. As discussed above, when Dr. David Jackson realized how intertwined his career was with the quality of his parenting, that gave him a whole new sense of commitment, energy, and resolve to enhance the quality of his career.

Get good at what you do

Career wellness involves being good at what you do, and having confidence that you can handle the job. Stress will always be a component of practicing law, but being confident in your abilities greatly reduces the chronic stress and feelings of being overwhelmed that plague many lawyers. This is one of the reasons why dissatisfaction among junior and associate lawyers is so high: The learning curve at the start of your law career is pretty much vertical. Everything is new. That is also why I don't recommend that any lawyer quit practicing within the first two years, unless there are immediate health or family concerns that must be dealt with. You need at least two years to get any sense of footing and to see what areas of law might best suit your interests and abilities.

Of course, it's easier to get good at what you do if you really enjoy what you do or why you do it; the two go hand-in-hand. To me, it comes down to this: If you produce good work and you're a good person, you give yourself much more latitude to create and enforce boundaries around your career commitments that will be respected by your superiors, colleagues, and clients. Quality of work is infinitely more important than quantity of work. For lawyers concerned about losing their jobs in the current climate of downsizing, office closures, and layoffs, lower your stress level by controlling what you can control: the quality of your work and the quality of your interactions with others. If you do good work and you're a good person and your firm still kicks you to the curb, well, you probably shouldn't be at that firm anyway. Even though it might not seem like it at the time, in the long run they're really doing you a favor.

Manage non-career stress

Another note about the interconnection of all dimensions of life is warranted here. Practicing law is stressful enough without bringing a bucketful of non-career stress with you to work every day. As I have discussed elsewhere in this book, stress in your marriage, with your health, with your kids, with your finances, or with your friends or extended family will show up as stress in your career, too. It will pack on top of the typical career stress and create a real and palpable sense of anxiety in your career. This can lead to depression, drug and alcohol dependency and addiction, and eventually to thoughts of suicide. Much has been written about this, including an entire book by Harvey Hyman, J.D. called *The Upward Spiral: Getting Lawyers from Daily Misery to Lifetime Wellbeing*.[91] When you're stressed, anxious, or overwhelmed at work, it becomes impossible to be an effective lawyer. The quality of your work suffers, creating more stress, and the vicious cycle continues. That is, again, why your holistic life plan is essential to your career, as it will greatly reduce the likelihood that you'll experience significant amounts of negative stress in other areas of life that will impact the quality of your lawyering.

Time management and technology

Time management and technology are two big factors that will not only impact your career wellness, but also the manner in which your career wellness will impact the other dimensions of your life. Much has been written about these issues and I won't go into them in detail here. Different tricks work for different people; there is no universal template. But I do want to make some comments about email, because your relationship with your inbox can have a huge impact on your career wellness and on your overall life.

Lots of people suggest checking emails and voicemails only at specific times of the day, and I know some lawyers that are able to stick to that with some regularity. I think that works well on some days. But the unpredictability of practicing law is what brings the excitement to it. No two days are ever the same, and that type of schedule doesn't fit well with structured and overly rigid routines for checking e-communications. I think it's a goal to work towards, but we shouldn't beat ourselves up if we can't stick to it entirely. At the same time, don't check every five minutes either. That's a recipe for disaster. The problem is, you might still get lots of time down on your sheet (if you're a super diligent recorder of time), but it's just not an efficient way of lawyering and will add to overall stress even if your billings don't suffer.

I practiced corporate and commercial law, and I remember well the barrage of emails in the last few days before a closing, most often with gigantic attachments containing redlined agreements, opinions, and closing documents. It was often overwhelming. *What do I review first? Who can I delegate to? Do we need a team meeting? Do we need a conference call? If so, is it just lawyers, or lawyers and clients? And what about the loan documents, when am I going to get to those? Where's the most recent version of the closing agenda anyway? No not the purchase agenda, the mezzanine financing agenda?* And so on.

If you're a commercial lawyer, I'm sure you can relate to this. Litigators and other lawyers hopefully can too. Your email is going to knock you off course every day. If you live by a daily to-do list, you know that your inbox will re-rewrite it for you—usually before you're finished your morning coffee. In many respects, that's just the nature of practice. The unpredictability of each day is what can make law exciting to practice. Overwhelming, sometimes, too.

There are two email best practices I'd like to share with you:

1. *Don't check email first thing in the morning.* Start the day on your own terms and get a good two hours of interruption-free work accomplished. That way, you can clear one or two high priority items off your list and get the momentum going for a good day. If you check your email first thing, you immediately switch into reaction mode, and often you'll find that none of your priority items get accomplished.

2. *Don't check your inbox unless you're prepared and able to deal with what you find there.* Think of it this way: What is the ratio of good news to bad news that comes in by regular mail? For me, it's mostly bills, unwanted fliers, and stuff someone else wants you to do. Rarely do you get a piece of mail that makes you say, *Awesome! Let's celebrate!*

   Is it any different with email? So why do we insist on checking it on Friday night or other times when we're not really working and have no intention of dealing with it right then anyway? What's the best that can come from it? You get an email saying you won a case or got a new client. Is that email going to be retracted between Tuesday at 9 p.m. and Wednesday at 9 a.m.? Will the feeling of happiness or elation caused by that email be any less when you ultimately do check it?

The more usual case is that you check email and it's something you don't want to see. Something that didn't turn out your way or that you have to deal with...but not right away. You've just compromised whatever free time you have by clogging your brain with stuff you're going to be glum about, stew over, or worry about—but not *do* anything about—for several hours.

Sometimes we check our inbox just to make sure nothing has come up that needs our attention. But if it *does* need your attention, are you going to do anything about it at that time? If not, don't check. Whatever good can come from it (and there's usually not much) can wait until later, and whatever bad that likely *will* come from it may ruin whatever non-work time you've tried to carve out for yourself. As Tim Ferriss writes, "Is your weekend really free if you find a crisis in your inbox Saturday morning that you can't address until Monday morning? Even if the inbox scan lasts 30 seconds, the preoccupation and forward projection for the subsequent 48 hours effectively deletes that experience from your life. You had time but you didn't have attention, so the time had no practical value."[92]

Pay attention to your work while you're working, and pay attention to whatever it is you do when you're not working while you're doing whatever it is you do when you're not working. Sounds kind of funny, but it's essential to experiencing health and vitality in your life. As Avner Offer said, "Attention is the universal currency of well-being."[93]

EMOTIONAL WELLNESS

Lawyers who disregard the importance that emotions play in their career and overall lives do so at their peril. After looking at the role of evolution, neuroscience, and other factors that affect happiness, *The Happy Lawyer* authors concluded that, "We are, at bottom, and to the disappointment of some, still much more emotional creatures than we are intellectual creatures."[94] Still, many lawyers fail to understand not only the importance of emotions, but the degree of control we have over our emotional intelligence.

In a recent survey conducted by Jordan Furlong of Law 21, respondents rated emotional intelligence the No. 1 feature with which to equip a future law firm—ahead of integrity, legal knowledge, innovation, and a host of other options.[95] Consequently, if you want to be an effective lawyer in tomorrow's legal landscape (not to mention today's) you need to pay attention to your ability to create, control, and express your emotions. This not only helps you foster great, lasting relationships with your clients, it helps you to be more effective in servicing those relationships as well. As Richard Susskind writes, in the future "it will not be sufficient for lawyers to be in possession of fine legal minds. Tomorrow's lawyers will need to acquire various softer skills if they are to win new clients and keep them happy."

When you bring a high level of stress to work with you, it causes you to feel overwhelmed and not in control. When you feel that way, it impacts how you act and the things you say. It affects your body language and the energy that emanates from you. Who wants to be around someone who is super-stressed, anxious, and unhappy? Or worse, someone who says and does mean, nasty, and malicious things, because they've let their emotions hot-wire their conscious brain? I don't care how smart you are, how brilliantly you can cross-examine a witness, or how cunningly you can achieve a settlement; if you're negative, chronically-stressed, and mean, I don't want to work with you and I certainly don't want to hire you. And apparently the respondents to the Law 21 survey don't want to, either.

Creating and controlling your emotions

The good news for those of you who struggle in this dimension of your life is that you can do things to enhance your emotional intelligence. You have a much greater degree of control over your daily emotions than you might think. No, you can't control every emotion that invades your being, good or bad, but you *can* do more of the things that create positive emotions, and do less of the things that create negative emotions. It starts with getting conscious about where your emotions come from and what causes them, and putting some habits in place to tilt your emotional scale much further towards positive emotions like joy, love, excitement, and happiness, than negative emotions like stress, panic, and boredom.

Creating a high level of emotional intelligence requires understanding that the Law of Cause and Effect applies to emotions, too. Our emotions are an effect of the circumstances that caused them. Create more circumstances that cause the effect of positive emotions, and you will experience more positive emotions. In other words, don't search for happiness head-on; achieve it by creating the circumstances that cause you to experience happiness. As Jon Stuart Mill said, "happiness should be approached sideways like a crab."[96]

For example, if you're a parent of young children, you probably know how stressful it can be to get the kids dressed, washed, fed, and to school on time. Hopefully without forgetting their bag, lunch, sneakers, homework and whatever else they need for school, too. As a result of the chaos of weekday mornings in my house, I often start my workday half-flustered, maybe a little grumpy, and often a little later than I had planned. That affects the quality of my work until I can get my head on straight again. But when I'm able to plan ahead a little bit, have the lunches and clean clothes ready, know where everyone's shoes are, and handle other little details that can make a big difference, the morning tends to go a little smoother, and the day starts out on a better emotional footing.

Here's an example that relates more to your work as a lawyer. Perhaps you have an assistant who's struggling to meet the demands of the job. She keeps making the same mistakes and it's driving you crazy. You're frustrated and irritated, and it's affecting not only your mood, but your work, too. It happens day after day. But the thing is, you're busy—really busy. Do you nevertheless find the time to train her properly, or, if it's a total lost cause, to find a replacement? Or do you use your "busyness" as an excuse to continue to suffer the negative emotional consequences of the working relationship?

These two examples relate to things you can do to avoid experiencing repeated negative emotions. As an example of how you might create positive emotions, think of a weekly date night habit with your spouse. If your weekly date is set for Wednesday nights, you're probably going to spend a lot of the day Wednesday happy, excited, and looking forward to that night. The sitter has been booked, the dinner reservations made, your new jacket is hanging in your closet. All that's left is to enjoy a great evening connecting with your spouse. That's a fool-proof formula for putting me in a great mood, and I bet it's the same for you.

It bears repeating here that regular exercise and proper nutrition also play a role in improving your emotional intelligence, since each helps you process and dissipate stress more efficiently. Going for a workout doesn't just clear your mind—it can clear out some negative emotions, too.

Controlling your response to circumstances beyond your control

In the course of your life, you'll suffer heartache and tragedies— hopefully few and far between—for which the only remedy will be time and as much positive energy as you can muster. But it is essential to always keep in mind that you *can* control how you react to life's circumstances that are beyond your control. For example, incivility among lawyers has become a growing concern in the profession. More and more, lawyers are treating each other without respect and courtesy—sometimes with outright malice— for the supposed purpose of gaining an advantage for their clients. You can't control how other lawyers treat you, but you can control the degree to which their conduct irritates you. You can choose to kill them with kindness. You can choose to realize the degree to which they must be suffering in one or more dimensions of their lives in order for them to think that acting with such incivility is acceptable. You can say a prayer for them, because even though their verbal abuse is directed at you, you know they must be in a very bad place to resort to such behavior. Be grateful you're not in such a place, and move on.

Expressing gratitude

If I only got to pick one best practice to improve my emotional wellness, it would be to express and exude gratitude on a daily basis. When something doesn't go your way, why not take a moment to take some deep breaths and think about all of the things in your life for which you are grateful—there are a ton of them. The coolest thing about gratitude is that you can't be pissed off and grateful at the same time. Gratitude trumps all. Yes, you still may have to deal with whatever angered you, but if you do it with feelings of gratitude, it will take a lot less out of you and you'll feel a whole lot better a lot more often. For further reading on this best practice, refer to the article called "Gratitude shuts the door on stress" in the Best of the Blog section of this book.

SPIRITUAL WELLNESS

First of all, let's demystify the concept of spirituality for those new to or skeptical of the term (I used to be one them). As with the concept of wellness, two lawyers could talk for an hour about spirituality and not even be talking about the same thing. Spirituality is not religion, it's not faith, and it's not prayer. Each of these may be ways to express or experience spirituality, but they are not synonymous with it.

Spirituality is where the big questions of life reside. *Why am I here? What's my place in this universe? What's my purpose on this planet?* Spirituality is the recognition that not everything in this universe can be explained by modern science; that there are profound elements at play in each of our lives that go beyond metrics and data. Your degree of wellness in the spiritual dimension of your life will have a greater impact on your level of fulfillment—and possibly your level of happiness, too—than perhaps any other dimension of life. It's pretty important stuff.

Finding your purpose

A few years ago, around the time I created my corporate wellness chart, I wasn't fulfilled in my life—which impacted my level of happiness—and I set out to figure out why. I had always believed that I had a role to play in the world, that I was put on this planet to make some kind of positive impact on it, and to leave it a better place than when I found it—not in an eradicate poverty or secure world peace kind of way, but more of an I want to fulfill my potential kind of way. I was spending a lot of time and thought trying to figure out my purpose in life and I was also trying to wrap my head around the concept of spirituality. I knew it was important, since all of the great teachers and authors I was reading said so—but I didn't really know what it was or how it was supposed to show up in my life. Initially I didn't include a division for spirituality in my corporate wellness chart, even though I knew it was important, because I really didn't know what it meant.

I thought that my purpose in life had to be driven by my career; in other words, I thought that the principal vehicle through which my purpose in life (once I discovered it) would manifest would be through my job. Since I didn't love practicing law, defining my life purpose in career terms was proving to be very difficult. I was stuck.

Within a couple of months, things clicked together. I listened to an audio interview in which Lifebook founder Jon Butcher described his life purpose. It was so simple and it passed by so quickly that I had to go back and listen to it again. And then again. I knew within minutes that it was my purpose too: *To create the highest possible quality of life for myself and my loved ones, and to help others do the same.* That was it. For me, that one sentence sums up the end game of why I'm on this planet. It's all about quality of life—not just having it, but *creating* it. And not just for me, but for my family and for others around me, too.

This is a purpose that can be lived throughout all dimensions of my life, not just in my career. Exercise, eating right, and meditating improves my quality of life. Spending time with my wife, kids, parents, brothers and their families, and with great friends...all of this improves my quality of life—and hopefully theirs, too. These days, my purpose plays out in my career as well, since I get to share information and lessons learned with lawyers around the world to help them achieve a higher quality of life. Indeed, writing this book has been an expression of my purpose.

But at the time I discovered this purpose, I was still practicing law, and so I got clear really quickly on how my work as a corporate and commercial lawyer improved quality of life for me, my family, and those around me. For my family and I, it was simple, as it was the means of providing the financial resources to pay for our desired standard of living—all within a wellness lifestyle, of course. But how did advising clients on business issues serve my purpose? At first I couldn't put it together—after all, I wasn't doing pro bono work all day. I wasn't defending people's human rights. I wasn't saving the environment. But then it hit me that what I did, and what all lawyers do, is to help make their clients' lives better, even if it's just a little bit at a time. The whole reason why a lawyer gets retained in the first place is that the client needs something done, but doesn't have the time, desire, or expertise to do it themselves. They need help.

If you've ever needed help with anything and received that help, what happened to your quality of life? It got better—if for an instant, a day, a year, or for life—it got better. Yes, this even applies to lawyers who act for big business all day long. Our world needs big business. Big business creates a ton of value. Industry has raised the quality of life in profound ways for most of the inhabitants of our planet over the last 200 years. Big business isn't perfect—not by a long shot—but it does in most cases move our quality of life forward. So if you're a lawyer for big business and you help them take care of their needs, you improve the quality of life of others, too.

I had found my purpose, but I still hadn't cracked the code on spirituality. Then, during my initial Lifebook lifestyle design session, I learned that living one's purpose in life is one of the main ways that a person can express and experience spirituality. Knowing your life's purpose essentially answers the question *Why am I here?* It's an incredibly grounding and fulfilling thing to have figured out. And finding ways to live your purpose on a daily basis? Well, for me, that's the crux of a spiritual life. In Maslow's terms, it's a quest for ever-increasing levels of self-actualization; it's the path towards being what I can be.

It was a tremendously powerful moment for me to put this all together. To realize that the two supposedly separate links to my missing fulfillment in life had come together and closed a loop was pretty special, to say the least. I cried. (My wife would probably say that I sobbed; she was in disbelief.) It was one of the few Eureka moments I have ever experienced—and it was wonderful.

What is your purpose? Why are you here? If you don't know, this book probably won't be able to provide the answers for you. I would simply encourage you to give it some thought, knowing that your career purpose and your greater life purpose don't have to be one and the same—although they should be congruent. And don't force it; the journey towards finding your purpose often plays an essential role in discovering it. Enjoy that journey.

Other expressions of spirituality

Finding and living one's life purpose isn't the only element of spirituality; there are certainly other wonderful ways in which to feel spiritually connected and to express your spirituality. For many, practicing their faith or religion is a way to do so. For other people, it's found in the service of others. For me, spirituality is expressed whenever you feel most alive—whenever you are experiencing a high level of vitality in your life.

Spending time in nature and connecting with the oneness of the universe can be a spiritual experience for some people. In this respect, there can be a spiritual component to fully understanding and adopting the wellness and prevention paradigm. That is, the concept that Nature intended us to be well and to express health, that we are all self-healing and self-regulating organisms, and that our bodies and minds will express health if given the essential nutrients and building blocks to do so. The wellness and prevention paradigm is a compelling example of the nexus of spirituality and science.

What kind of world will we build?

There's a wonderful phrase in *The Happy Lawyer* about the purpose that lawyers play in society. The phrase is simply, "Lawyers help build the world."[97] It's an idea straight out of the mind of Ayn Rand.

In our work as lawyers, we provide such an essential and immeasurable service to society that we do, in fact, help build the world. It's an idea that makes me proud to be a lawyer—and it should make you proud, too.

But what *kind* of world will we build? What will be its *quality*? Think back for a moment to the discussion on genetics in Chapter 3, about the fact that your genetic blueprint doesn't determine your degree of health, happiness, and fulfillment any more than an architect's blueprint determines the quality of the building that it depicts. In each case, the blueprint is the starting point, but the real determinants of the outcome are the inputs used to create it. If we, as lawyers, help build the world, then it will be, in part, *our* craftsmanship that determines the quality of the world that is built.

Will we live a wellness lifestyle that produces the raw materials—health, happiness, and fulfillment—we will require to be effective in this task?

A healthier legal services profession will help build a healthier world. But our profession will only become healthier if the lawyers who are members of it become healthier, too.

What will you choose?

BEST OF THE BLOG

SELECTED THOUGHTS FROM
THE WELLNESS LAWYER BLOG
@ www.wellnesslawyer.com

10 steps to start your day with exercise

Many lawyers find it difficult to find time to exercise. The best way to ensure you get regular exercise is to work out in the morning before you start your day. I'm sure you've heard this a million times. It sounds great in theory, but theory tends to be sleeping when the alarm goes off in the morning! So you need more than theory. You need an action plan.

Here it is:

Wellness Lawyer's 10-step action plan to wake up to exercise (and wake up to your life!).

1. Before you go to bed at night, set out your work out clothes. *Ok,* you say, *I can do that.*
2. Whatever time you currently get up in the morning, get up an hour earlier. *An hour earlier? Are you crazy? I don't get enough sleep as it is!*
3. Seriously, get up an hour earlier. If that means setting your alarm for an hour and a half earlier that's fine—that way you still get to hit snooze for a half hour. *An hour AND A HALF earlier? Didn't he hear what I just said? I need my sleep!*
4. Set the alarm on the other side of the room if you have to. Set it to music that will make you want to yak (*eg.* Celine

Dion) to ensure you won't be able to get back to sleep. *Yikes! That WOULD make me want to yak.*

5. After yaking, put your work out clothes on. *Still thinking of waking up to Celine Dion. I'm a little queasy. Give me a minute.*

6. Work out. Go for a walk. Go for a jog. Go for a run. Do yoga. Ride your bike. Do a workout DVD. Lift some weights. Whatever it is you want to do, do it for 30 minutes. *I suppose I could try that DVD I got for my birthday, or maybe give my bike a try to see if it still works.*

7. When you're done, you'll notice that you're probably the only one up in your house. Quiet huh? And you'll notice that you're full of sweat and fully awake and it's still 20-30 minutes before you're normally up. *I guess that would be sorta cool.*

8. Reward yourself by spending that time however you want. Have a long shower. Read the paper. Have a leisurely breakfast, maybe even eat some real food. Do some online shopping. Tidy up those unwieldy nose hairs. Whatever you want—you've earned it. *I'll probably just want to go back to sleep. But now that you mention it, my nose hairs could use some trimming.*

9. Pay attention to how you feel the rest of the day. See if any of these words and phrases come to mind: **Calmer. Less stressed. More alert.** A little sore, maybe, but in a good way. **More energy**—more than enough to snicker audibly each time a colleague mentions how busy they are and how they'll have to skip their workout again today. *Wow, I'd take even just one of those phrases. And it WOULD be fun to stick it to Collins and Bannerman who always bring their gym bag and never work out.*

10. Have a great night's sleep. (You won't have to work at this one, it'll just happen.) *I don't doubt it. After getting up an hour earlier I'll probably be lights out before the kids!*

11. Do it all again. **Make it a habit.** Pretty soon it'll just be part of who you are. And you won't even need Celine to get you out of bed. *Now wait a second. You mean I have to do this more than once? And by the way, why should I listen to you—you can't even count! Some 10-step plan this is!*

True, my counting skills may need some work, but the long and the short of it is this: Give up one hour's sleep and the other 23 hours of your day will be better. Or sleep an extra hour and compromise the quality of the other 23 hours of the day.

As with everything in life, the choice is yours.

***

How do you slow...down...time?

Lawyers, more than most people, often struggle to find enough time in the day to get everything done. But I don't think that's such a bad thing. It's a sign that you're motivated and driven and take pride in your work and in the rest of your life, and you want to get the most out of it.

What *is* a bad thing in my opinion is when someone looks back at a period of time (ie. a month, or a year) and thinks *Geez... where did all the time go?*

To me, that's a sign of not **living consciously**. It's a sign of not living in the moment enough and of not being present enough with what you're doing and how you're feeling.

If you look back on the last month or year and say it was all a blur, then you have not been focused enough on living your life. You've probably been too focused on what comes next rather than what is now.

Don't get me wrong. It is important to think about and plan for the future, no question. But the future is a process. **Your *life* is a process.** You have to take notice of, and enjoy, the process.

You need to **enjoy the now**—not to the detriment of the future, but to the betterment of the future.

Enjoying the now doesn't mean eating chocolate cake every day and maxing out credit cards. Enjoying the now means enjoying the process of living and working towards a life of happiness and fulfillment.

Enjoying the now means taking notice of the things that make you happy, and of the things that don't make you happy, so that you can work to create more of the happy and less of the unhappy in the future.

Enjoying the now means EXPERIENCING your life. Tasting it, savouring it—like you would a fine wine.

When you do that, you will be bringing an increased level of consciousness to your life. **And when you bring increasing consciousness to your life, TIME SLOWS DOWN.**

Now, you might say, *Yeah but as the old saying goes, time flies when you're having fun. So if time slows down, you must not be having fun!*

Well, I've got two responses for that. First, it's just an old saying. Maybe it's time to throw it out, and replace it with *Time flies when you're not paying attention to your life.*

Second, I think that saying is meant to apply only to short periods of time—like a night out with friends, for example. I know that when my wife and I get a babysitter and get out with friends—or better yet, a date night for just the two of us—the clock really seems to race by no matter how conscious I am to make sure I enjoy every moment of it.

Frankly, I think that people for whom large periods of time (weeks, months, years) "fly by" subconsciously *want* them to fly by—because they're simply not enjoying the process of experiencing their life. They're not leading happy, fulfilled lives. They've chosen to turn the autopilot light on and to keep it on.

If you're one of those people, **it's time to turn off the autopilot and to start *experiencing* your life.**

I've been on autopilot before and let me tell you, living consciously is a lot more fun. You feel so much more *alive!*

You have to work at it, but it›s worth it. Because **living consciously will buy you what money can't: TIME.**

***

Affirmations can make you a hero

Affirmations are an excellent way to get your day off to a great start. They help get you in the proper frame of mind and give you a better chance of having the kind of day you want to have, rather than the kind of day that just happens to you.

If you're new to affirmations, they're simply things you say to yourself that you like to hear, that you believe (or want to believe) about yourself, and that keep you focused on what's important to you.

For example, here are some excerpts of my daily affirmation:

My life works PERFECTLY.

Today is a GIFT for which I am SO GRATEFUL. I am SO EXCITED to start this day.

Today I will be FULL OF ENERGY. I will BE FIT, EAT RIGHT, and THINK WELL.

Today I will LIVE MY PURPOSE, which is to create an EPIC QUALITY OF LIFE for me and my family and to help others do the same. An epic quality of life, to me, means a life of SIMPLICITY and STRESS-FREE ABUNDANCE.

Today I will be a GREAT HUSBAND. Today Shelley will know that SHE COMES FIRST.

Today I will be a GREAT DAD to Alex, Gabe and Noah. I will enrich their lives today.

Affirmations can be a few words, or a sentence, a paragraph or a whole page—several pages even. Mine's about a page long. As you can see, I like to capitalize the key terms of my affirmation so that they pop out at me when I read them—these are the things that I really want to emphasize. These are the touchstones of my life that I always want to be in my consciousness.

I have been in the off-and-on routine of daily affirmations for about a year and a half now. I haven't quite made them a habit yet, but one of my goals for January is to do just that—to make it a priority to say my affirmations out loud, with feeling, every morning.

Now at first you can feel sort of silly doing this—I'm still getting used to it myself. Until today, I had always said my affirmations alone, either in the morning before anyone else is up, or in the shower, or while driving in the car.

But this morning (the first morning back to school for the kids) I just started blurting them out while the kids were having breakfast. At first they just listened and looked at each other as if to say, Dad's being weird again. Then after a couple of my affirmations, my 5 year-old Gabriel said "Me too", as in Today I will be FULL OF ENERGY ("Me too!") I will BE FIT, EAT RIGHT, and THINK WELL ("Me too!").

Then when I got to the part about being a GREAT DAD they all cheered. It was awesome. So I just kept going, and the kids kept cheering, and when I was done my 7 year-old Alexandra said, "Dad, you're talking like Sensei Wu today."

For the uninitiated, Sensei Wu is the wise old mentor of the 4 Lego Ninjago ninjas, who have become de facto members of our family. So to be compared to the highly revered sensei was basically like being called a hero. By my kids. Over breakfast.

How cool is that?

So be a hero. Get your affirmations together and then just blast them out in front of your family one day. See what happens. I'd love to hear all about it.

✳✳✳

Vacations are the perfect reminder why a wellness lifestyle matters

Just back from a wonderful family vacation in the beautiful province of Newfoundland & Labrador (Canada's eastern-most province). It is my wife Shelley's home province, and it is not always known for having the best weather—even in summer. We lucked out this year. The weather was almost tropical at times. Add to that the breathtaking coastlines and vistas, and I had to catch myself once or twice from thinking we were vacationing in the Greek Islands or the South Pacific. (Might have been the Screech!)

Shelley and I caught ourselves thinking a few times during our vacation just how lucky were are to have a quality of life that allows us to travel to great places and to spend time with friends and family.

Shelley and I discussed a few times during our trip how it was precisely those kind of experiences that enrich our lives in a profound way, and that we wanted to have tons more great vacations with the kids to places all over the globe—not to mention some adult-only trips!

I bring all of this up because our Newfoundland vacation reminded us that **one of the key purposes behind our commitment to leading a healthy lifestyle is so that we are physically able to have wonderful vacation and travel experiences for years to come.** And I'm not talking about five or ten years here—I'm talking about forty or fifty! We're in our late 30s now. We want to be continuing to have these great experiences when we're in our 80s and 90s!

But we know that won't be possible unless we commit ourselves TODAY to living a healthy lifestyle. Our motto is Be Fit, Eat Right, Think Well, Get Adjusted, and we try to live that every day. Sure there are some days that we stray a little from our target. Vacation eating tends to be a little wayward. But how can you resist the temptation of a perfectly crafted Smore?

The main thing is that we realize that we have to do the right things *today* to have those great experiences for years to come.

We have other compelling purposes that propel our commitment to wellness living, including serving as healthy role models for our three children. But vacations and travel experiences spent with family are probably the most tangible things that remind us of the IMMENSE value and reward for making healthy choices every day.

So what about you? **What are *your* most compelling purposes that drive your commitment to wellness living?** Writing them down and sharing them publicly will help propel you in the direction you choose, so please feel free to share them with our readers by leaving a comment below.

Until next time. . .Be Well, Live your Purpose, Love your Life!

***

The best time to plant a tree

I absolutely LOVE this old proverb:

> *"The best time to plant a tree is 20 years ago. The second best time is now."*

I think it's the perfect concept for those who procrastinate on their health and wellness goals—and for those who justify not setting any.

How many times have you heard someone say something like "I wish I'd have done that years ago", or "If only I'd started that when I was in my 20s", or some variation of that theme.

Well, you may be able to slow down time, but as far as I know there's no way to turn it back.

People often use the fact that they didn't do or know something in the past as a reason or excuse or justification for not doing or changing something in the future.

Let's look at eating organic foods, for example. When faced with the choice of buying and eating organic vs. non-organic foods, some people say "Well, I never ate organic growing up, and I turned out okay—and besides, the damage, if there is any, is already done. Why change now?"

The same applies for taking quality nutritional supplements like Omega 3, Vitamin D and probiotics, or for getting regular chiropractic adjustments, or for just plain getting some regular exercise. Heck, it even applies to changing careers if you don't love the one you're in.

Changing something now doesn't mean that you were wrong or stupid or lazy in the past. We've all made tons of mistakes and we've all done dumb things (and *not* done smart things) in our lives.

But NOT changing something now when you know it's good for you just because you didn't do it in the past—well, that is wrong and stupid and lazy.

Yes, many of us wish that 20 years ago we started saving 10% of every paycheque…and started exercising regularly…and eating whole foods…and not eating processed foods…and had chosen the right career...and planned a little better for the future...and the list goes on.

Twenty years ago definitely would have been the best time to do all of this. But, as the proverb says, the second best time is NOW.

So get out of your own way and get on with those changes you know you need to make to improve your overall level of wellness and quality of life. Twenty years from now you'll be happy you did.

***

Lawyer + commitment to wellness = 95 lost pounds

Many lawyers might think that the pursuit of wellness sounds great in theory but just don't have the time to put much into it. After all, we work long hours and our client obligations never seem to cease. And it's our clients who pay the bills, so we can't leave them out of earshot while we head off to get some exercise, right?

Let me share with you a story that might change your mind. Maurice Chiasson was a colleague of mine at Stewart McKelvey. Maurice has a busy corporate and commercial practice and significant volunteer commitments. He's a QC and he works over 2,000 hours per year.

Three plus years ago, Maurice weighed 287 pounds. He was on high blood pressure meds. He knew that it would probably be a good idea to shed a few pounds, and tried off and on to get active, but life got in the way and he couldn't get committed to it.

Then one day Maurice walked up 4 flights of stairs to attend a meeting on another floor of the office. When he got to the meeting he was completely winded and had to take a few moments to recover. He realized then and there that he had to do something—for real this time—about his health. He was 43 years old at the time and thought to himself *if I don't do something about this, I'm not going to see 50.*

So he did do something. He decided to apply to his pursuit of better health the same level of commitment he had always brought to serving his clients. He hired a personal trainer and considered every workout as a meeting with himself—a meeting he would no more cancel than if it were a meeting with one of his clients.

That said, Maurice eased into his exercise routine. To his credit, he did not try to go from zero to P90X in one fell swoop. He began with light workouts 3 times a week. Over the span of two years he gradually progressed to high impact workouts five times a week. And he has added a focus on proper nutrition to his pursuit of wellness.

Maurice acknowledges that there were a few plateaus along the way, but **two years after his fateful flight up the Stewart McKelvey stairwells, Maurice had lost 95 pounds!**

And better yet, no more meds!

Only two years before, Maurice's medical doctor had suggested that due to his family history Maurice would probably be on high blood pressure meds for the rest of his life. **It's not heredity that controls our wellness, folks. It's our choices, it's how we live our lives**—our level of commitment, as Maurice might say.

Nowadays, Maurice says he couldn't imagine not exercising regularly and eating right. If he goes a couple of days without exercising, his body starts to crave the endorphins the body creates when engaged in physical activity. *It's addictive,* he says. *Addicted to wellness*—**what an awesome concept.**

So, do you still think you're too busy to make wellness a priority in your life?

Can you really afford not to?

***

Work/life balance? What a bunch of crap.

My mom always told me never to use the word hate. "It's such a strong word," she used to say. "Use something different, like *loathe*."

And my 6-year old daughter obviously picked up the same message in Grade 1. "Dad!" she exclaims whenever I use the H-word. "You shouldn't say that word. It's not nice!"

Well, with apologies to my mother and my daughter, I have to say that I HATE the phrase *work/life balance*. What a bunch of crap.

Whenever I hear it my ears hurt a little bit. Whenever I read it I squint painfully, in much the same way a man does when they see another man get hit in the groin with a flying object.

Let me explain why this combination of words irritates me so much. It's only three words and a slash, after all. You'd think I could just let it go.

Regrettably, I cannot.

I get the *balance* bit. That part I'm okay with. It fits with wellnesslawyer.com's philosophy that there are lots of divisions or categories in one's life that need attention and need to be worked on and nurtured in order to maximize one's wellness and quality of life.

It's the *work/life* part that makes me want to vomit a little bit.

It appears to me that the proponents of the phrase *work/life balance* are trying to articulate that Work and Life should be in some sort of balance.

The way I see it, there's only one problem with this. **Work and Life <u>are not</u> two separate, mutually exclusive things! Work is *a part* of life. Work is *one component* of life.**

The phrase *work/life balance* makes it seem like there's Work, and then there's Everything Else in Life, and as long as Everything Else in Life is of equal weight to our Work, then we should get some sort of medal under the Weights and Measures Act!

Trying to balance Work and Life is like trying to balance one body part with your entire body. What weighs more, your kidney or your whole body?

If it's work/life balance that you seek, you'll never get there because it's simply impossible. You're starting from the premise that your Work is separate from your Life and/or that your Work should be equal to the rest of your Life. Both premises are wrong! And when you start from a faulty premise, you have no chance of reaching your destination.

You have one life. It is made up of tons of things—some important and some not so much. **Yes, work is a very important part of life. *But it is only a part of your life.*** It deserves tons of attention but so do your family, your finances, your friends, your spirituality, your philanthropy, your health, your intellect and your mindset. The list could go on.

So please help me in banishing the phrase *work/life balance* from the English language. Let's dump it in the scrap heap with other outdated and harmful phrases like *would you like fries with that?* and *pass the remote.*

***

Too busy to get to the gym? Try this.

Let's face it: for many lawyers the prospect of getting to the gym everyday, or even on a semi-regular basis, is not great. We're busy, usually *really* busy, so with work and family and the commute and the non-profit board meeting and the dentist appointment and . . . who has time to get to the gym?

It takes 10 minutes to get there, 5 minutes to change, 5 minutes to stretch, 30 minutes on the treadmill, 20 minutes lifting a few weights, 5 minutes for some abs, 5 minutes for some idle chatter, 15 minutes to shower and get dressed, and 10 minutes to get back to the office. And that's if you don't have to wait around for vacant equipment!

You can check my math, but by my count that's an hour and forty-five minutes door to door to get your workout in. For most of us in the billable hour world, that's just not sustainable.

We know we'd feel better if we worked out, but most days we just can't fit it in. And then not only do we not get the benefit of a workout, we also feel bad that we didn't work out, so it's a double whammy. It's not long before that begins to take its toll on us.

What if you could get the same workout in 45 minutes or less, including changing and showering? Would you be more inclined to make some time in your day for it?

If so, you should pick up a copy of Jillian Michael's 30 Day Shred DVD.

In a word, it's awesome. The workout is only 18 minutes, with a few minutes of warm up and cool down stretching on top of that, so about 25 minutes in total. It combines cardio and strength training with some abs to boot. There's no downtime in the workout, so it's not the most pleasant 18 minutes you'll spend all day, but when you're finished, you'll feel like you just worked out hard for an hour and you'll have an extra jump in your step the rest of the day.

There's three levels to choose from, and you can always increase or decrease your hand weights to adjust the difficulty of the workout. Try it every other day for a month and you will notice a difference in your body, your energy levels, and your overall wellness, guaranteed.

For all you guys out there who are saying exercise DVDs are for girls, well, you may be right. But if it saves me an hour a day and makes it exponentially more likely that I'll get my workout in on a regular basis, then I say *pass me my leg warmers, where do I sign up?*

(Believe me, I was skeptical at first too. Last summer when my wife Shelley brought home the DVD and asked me to try it with her, I didn't even bother to put shoes on because I thought it'd be such a breeze. The next day I could barely walk.)

So if getting to the gym regularly is a problem for you, then get the DVD, get up a half hour earlier and get your workout in before the rest of the family is awake. It's a killer way to start your day. If that doesn't work, bring it to the office, pop it in your computer and get your workout in at lunchtime. (You might want to shut the door). Hopefully you have a shower at the office because you <u>will</u> be sweating buckets. Or you could do it at night after the kids are in bed as a great way to relieve some of the stress that may have built up during the day.

It's up to you. But no more excuses that you don't have time to workout. I've just saved you an hour. And as we all know, in our business more than most, time is money.

***

Baby steps

Embarking on a path to wellness is not an all-or-nothing affair. I think a lot of people make this mistake. They think that they have to wake up one day and completely change their lives in order to achieve their wellness goals. Well, unless you're superman, that won't work. Change has to occur gradually. We have to learn new habits, and that takes time. It's not easy, that's for sure. So that's why, for us mere mortals, change needs to happen in small, manageable steps.

I have a 10 month old son. His name is Noah. He's our third child, so I should be used to it by now. But it's still amazing to watch him pick up new things every day. In the last month he's gone from stationary to wiggle to worm to commando crawl to hands and knees crawl and now he's pulling himself up to his feet to get a better glimpse of what big brother and sister are up to. It's been amazing to watch his progress—even though I've seen it twice before with my other kids, and even though it's the exact same process every other kid in the world goes through.

It's all about baby steps. Gradual change. Change that is almost imperceptible from day to day, but after a month or so it becomes remarkable. And once you build some momentum, it'll be harder to stop the change than to keep going on your path to wellness.

Fact is, everyday we make choices that take us closer to wellness or further away from it. We don't need to wake up one day and suddenly become fitness freaks, health food fanatics, spiritual zealots, and lawyer of the year material. But we do need to be conscious of the choices we make everyday. While at first we may not be able to make every choice a choice for wellness, we can certainly make some. Each day we can make more and more. And eventually our healthy choices will become second nature and we'll hardly recognize our former selves, the people we were before we made our commitment to choosing wellness.

Healthy choices. One at a time. So easy a baby can do it.

***

Cool lawyers drink green smoothies

One of the biggest improvements my wife and I have made with respect to healthy eating over the last year has been the addition of green smoothies to our morning routine. We had been drinking fruit smoothies off-and-on for a while before that, but moving towards more of a vegetable-based blend has been a big win for us in the diet department.

When you consume a blender full of nutrients in the morning, not only do you give yourself an energy boost, but an insurance policy of sorts as well: even if you eat like crap the rest of the day (not the game plan, but it happens) you're still guaranteed to have reached most, if not all, of your minimum recommended fruit and veggie intake for the day.

Here's a recipe you can try:
1 cup spinach
1 cup kale
3 celery sticks
½ medium-sized cucumber
½ avocado
6-8 large frozen strawberries
¼ cup frozen blueberries
½ banana
1 cup almond milk
½ cup pineapple juice
Vega or Manitoba Harvest protein powder (optional, but recommended if you work out in the morning or if you drink your smoothies as a meal replacement; check label for serving size)

It tastes great (I was a skeptic at first too), and pretty soon you'll find yourself craving vegetables in the morning!

***

Gratitude shuts the door on stress

Expressing and exuding GRATITUDE is one of the best ways to manage stress in your legal career and in your life. You've probably heard variations on this theme before, along the lines of "things could be worse so be thankful for what you've got."

But REALLY stepping into a mindset of gratitude goes much more than that. It's about literally pausing to reflect not only about what you HAVE, but also about the everyday wonders of the world all around you and about all of the people and experiences and circumstances that have brought you where you are today.

One really cool thing about gratitude that I learned from a mentor of mine is that **it's impossible to feel stress or anxiety (or any other negative emotion) while expressing gratitude**. In other words, when you are in a grateful frame of mind, you literally shut the door on stress.

This applies to exercise too. You know when you're working out and you're pushing yourself and it's starting to get a little painful (a good painful, but painful nonetheless)? In those moments, try expressing gratitude that your body can even ATTEMPT to do what it's doing, and I bet you'll find the pain lessens enough to get you through your workout.

This week, commit to taking a moment every day to express gratitude for FIVE people or things or experiences or whatever it is you might feel grateful for in that moment. Your best bet is to pick the SAME TIME each day for this, and to set a reminder for it in your calendar. It'll only take a couple of minutes each day. Many people find that gratitude sessions are a great way to start the day upon waking up, or a wonderful way to end the day just before bed. Pick what works best for you and stick to it.

And if you want to go all the way with this challenge, WRITE DOWN your five things each day. By the end of the week you'll have a list of over 30 items and you'll have started your very own Gratitude Journal.

✳✳✳

Does your office have a culture of wellness?

Most law offices these days offer wellness subsidies to their lawyers, and this is a good thing, no question. But subsidies should not be the be all and end all of a firm's wellness strategy. Firms that foster a **culture of wellness** will have greater success than those that simply throw money at the issue.

Here are two ways to know if your firm has a culture of wellness:

1. Do you feel any sense of professional guilt if you're seen leaving the office in the middle of the day with a gym bag over your shoulder? Do you get a sense that your colleagues applaud your commitment to working out, or that they mumble under their breath that you should be "working during work hours" (whatever that means!)? If you don't feel 100% free to work out when you want, then what good is the "free" gym membership your firm pays for anyway?

2. What kind of snacks does your firm keep around in the kitchen(s) of your office, either for free or for purchase? If you can walk down the hall and quickly grab a soda, or chips, or cookies or the like, then you don't have much of a culture of wellness in your office. Firms that provide or make available for purchase healthy snacks like raw fruit and vegetables, almonds, and high-quality organic or all-natural protein and energy bars, are the firms that have really thought through what it means to support its lawyers' levels of wellness.

This week, give some thought to whether or not your firm or office has a culture of wellness. Go for a workout in the middle of the day and get a sense of what your colleagues' reaction to this is. And have a look at the snacks made available in your office—does eating what's available improve your level of wellness or not? If you see some area where your firm could improve its culture of wellness, talk to your HR manager or wellness committee about it. And if that person is you—then take charge and improve your firm's culture of wellness this week.

NOTES

Introduction

[1]   There is even a blog called *101 Reasons to Kill All The Lawyers.* The kicker? It's written by a lawyer. www.101reasonstokillallth elawyers.com.

[2]   Canadian Bar Association, *Survey of Lawyers on Wellness Issues,* Legal Profession Assistance Conference, (2012).

[3]   University of New South Wales, *The Health and Well-being Survey of Australian Lawyers,* www.law.unsw.edu.au/wellbeing.

[4]   See for example, American Bar Association, *The Report of At the Breaking Point: A national conference on the emerging crisis in the quality of lawyers' health and lives—its impact on law firms and client services,* (1991), and ABA Young Lawyers Division, *Life in the Balance: Achieving equilibrium in professional and personal life,* (2002-2003).

[5]   Duke University School of Law Professor Daniel S. Bowling, III teaches a course called "Well-being and the Practice of Law", www.law.duke.edu/events/well-being-and-practice-law.

Chapter 1

[6]   Elwork, Amiran Ph.D., *Stress Management for Lawyers: How to Increase Personal and Professional Satisfaction in the Law,* 3rd ed., North Wales, PA: Vorkell Group, 2007, p. 7.

[7]   Schiltz, Patrick J., *On Being a Happy, Healthy, and Ethical Member of an Unhappy, Unhealthy, and Unethical Profession,* Vanderbilt Law Review, Vol. 52, 1999, p. 905.

8   Harper, Steven J., *The Lawyer Bubble: A Profession in Crisis*, New York: Basic Books, 2013, p. xiii.

9   Susskind, Richard, *Tomorrow's Lawyers: An Introduction to Your Future*, Oxford: Oxford University Press, 2013, p. 4.

Chapter 2

10   World Health Organization, www.who.int/hia/evidence/doh/en/.

11   *Ibid.*

12   Vanderbilt Law Review, Vol. 52, 1999, p. 881.

13   Levit, Nancy and Linder, Douglas O., *The Happy Lawyer: Making a Good Life in the Law*, New York: Oxford University Press, 2010, p. 6.

14   McMillan, Amanda, *Best and worst jobs for your health*, May 19, 2012, www.foxnews.com/health/2012/05/17/best-and-worst-jobs-for-your-health.

15   Canadian Bar Association, *Survey of Lawyers on Wellness Issues*, Legal Profession Assistance Conference, (2012).

16   *Ibid.*

17   Levit and Linder, *supra* note 13, p. 48

18   Levit and Linder note in *The Happy Lawyer*, *supra* note 13, p. 18, that there were more than 4,000 books published on the subject of happiness in 2008 alone.

19   Levit and Linder, *supra* note 13, p. 40.

20   *Ibid.*, p. 30, quoting neuroscientist Richard Davidson.

21   *Ibid.*, p. 25.

22   *Ibid.*, p. 38.

23   *Ibid.*, p. 10.

24   Butcher, Jon. *The Big Picture Principle*. Lifebook VIP membership page, September 2013.

25   Elwork, Amiran Ph.D., *Stress Management for Lawyers: How to Increase Personal and Professional Satisfaction in the law*, 3rd ed., North Wales, PA: Vorkell Group, 2007, p. 32.

26   Smith, Jacqueline, *The Happiest and Unhappiest Jobs in America*, Forbes.com, March 2013, *www.forbes.com/sites/jacquelynsmith/2013/03/22/the-happiest-and-unhappiest-jobs-in-america/*

[27]   Levit and Linder, *supra* note 13, p. 8.

[28]   *Ibid.*, p. 65.

[29]   Seligman, Martin E. P., Ph.D., *Why Are Lawyers so Unhappy?*, November 16, 2012, www.lawyerswithdepression.com/articles/why-are-lawyers-so-unhappy/

[30]   *Ibid.*

[31]   Levit and Linder, *supra* note 13, p. 44.

[32]   *Ibid.*, p. 45-6.

[33]   Johnson, Brian, *Philosopher's Note on* Motivation and Personality *by Abraham Maslow*, p. 2.

[34]   Melcher, Michael F., *The Creative Lawyer: A Practical Guide to Authentic Professional Satisfaction*, Chicago: American Bar Association, 2007, p. 9.

[35]   Latham, Tyger, Psy.D., *The Depressed Lawyer*, Psychology Today, May 2, 2011, www.psychologytoday.com/blog/therapy-matters/201105/the-depressed-lawyer.

[36]   Harper, Steven J., *The Lawyer Bubble: A Profession in Crisis*, New York: Basic Books, 2013, p. 60.

[37]   *Ibid.*, p. 63.

[38]   Dave Nee Foundation, *www.daveneefoundation.com/lawyers-and-depression*.

[39]   Harper, *supra* note 36, p. 57.

[40]   Levit and Linder, *supra* note 13, p. 221.

[41]   *Ibid.*, p. 52.

[42]   Harper, *supra* note 36, p. 58.

[43]   Chen, Vivia, *How Lawyers Rank in American Society*, The Careerist, July 18, 2013, *thecareerist.typepad.com/thecareerist/2013/07/miscel.html*.

Chapter 3

[44]   Chiropractic Leadership Alliance, *Infinite Wisdom: An Interview with Dr. Deepak Chopra*, Best of On Purpose, Vol. 4, CD 5.

[45]   Chestnut, James, D.C., *The Wellness & Prevention Paradigm*, audio summary, 2-CD set, 2012.

[46]   Lipton, Bruce H., Ph.D., *The Biology of Belief*, Santa Rosa, CA: Elite Books, 2005, p. 52.

[47]   *Ibid.*, p. 15.

48 Chestnut, *supra* note 45.

49 *Ibid.*

50 *Ibid.*

51 *Ibid.*

52 Chestnut, James, D.C., *The Wellness & Prevention Paradigm*, Victoria: The Wellness Practice—Global Self Health Corp., 2011, p. 47.

53 Lipton, *supra* note 46, p. 72.

54 Chestnut, *supra* note 45.

55 Lipton, *supra* note 46, p. 52.

Chapter 4

56 Gentempo, Patrick, D.C., *Foundations of Wellness*, audio series, Creating Wellness Alliance, *www.creatingwellness.com* (members portal).

57 *Be Fit. Eat Right. Think Well.* is the motto of the Creating Wellness Alliance.

58 Chestnut, James, D.C., *The Wellness & Prevention Paradigm*, Victoria: The Wellness Practice-Global Self Health Corp., 2011, p. 116.

59 Schiltz, Patrick J., *On Being a Happy, Healthy, and Ethical Member of an Unhappy, Unhealthy, and Unethical Profession*, Vanderbilt Law Review, Vol. 52, 1999, p. 910.

60 *Ibid.*, p. 937-938.

Chapter 5

61 Chestnut, James, D.C., *The Wellness & Prevention Paradigm*, Victoria: The Wellness Practice-Global Self Health Corp., 2011, p. 58.

62 Branden, Nathaniel, *The Six Pillars of Self-Esteem*, New York: Bantam, 1995, p. 143.

63 Melcher, Michael F., *The Creative Lawyer: A Practical Guide to Authentic Professional Satisfaction*, Chicago: American Bar Association, 2007, p. 3.

64 Harper, Steven J., *The Lawyer Bubble: A Profession in Crisis*, New York: Basic Books, 2013, p. xvi.

Chapter 6

65 Evans, Mike, M.D., *23 and ½ hours: What is the single best thing we can do for our health?*, *www.youtube.com/watch?v= aUaInS6HIGo*.

66 Levit, Nancy and Linder, Douglas O., *The Happy Lawyer: Making a Good Life in the Law*, New York: Oxford University Press, 2010, p. 30-1.

67 Ben-Shahar, Tal, *Cheer up. Here's how...*, The Guardian, December 29, 2007, www.theguardian.com/lifeandstyle/2007/ dec/29/healthandwellbeing.mentalhealth

68 Evans, *supra* note 65.

69 Horford, Patrick, *The Optimum Nutrition Bible*, London: Piatkus, 2004, p. 13.

70 Chestnut, James, D.C., *The Innate Diet & Natural Hygiene*, Victoria: The Wellness Practice—Global Self Health Corp., 2004, p. 32.

71 Cordain, Loren, Ph.D., *The Paleo Diet*, New York: John Wiley & Sons, Inc., 2002 (as quoted in Chestnut, *supra* note 70, p. 42).

72 Horford, *supra* note 69, p. 11.

73 Chestnut, *supra* note 70, p. 34.

74 Johnson, Brian, *Philosopher's Note on* Prevent and Reverse Heart Disease *by Caldwell B. Esselstyn, M.D.*, p.5.

75 Chestnut, *supra* note 70, p. 101

76 The source for all information in the section "Nutritional Supplements" is Chestnut, *Innate Choice: The Science of Wellness Nutrition*, www.innatechoice.com.

77 Horford, *supra* note 69, p. 253.

78 Lipton, Bruce H., Ph.D., *The Biology of Belief*, Santa Rosa, CA: Elite Books, 2005, p. 108.

79 *Medical Errors, The FDA, and Problems with Prescription Drugs*, www.cancure.org/medical_errors.htm.

80 Hyman, Harvey, J.D., *The Upward Spiral: Getting Lawyers from Daily Misery to Lifetime Wellbeing*, Piedmont, CA: Lawyers' Wellbeing, Inc., 2010, p. 294.

81 Levit and Linder, *supra* note 66, p. 30.

[82] Brian Johnson interview with Jon Butcher, Lifebook VIP membership page, May 2013.
[83] In fact, I used to confuse it with *levitation*. I thought meditators sat cross-legged and actually rose off the ground, levitation-style. Seriously.

Chapter 7

[84] Levit, Nancy and Linder, Douglas O., *The Happy Lawyer: Making a Good Life in the Law*, New York: Oxford University Press, 2010, p. 236.
[85] *Ibid.*, p. 90.
[86] *Ibid.*, p. 37.
[87] Ferriss, Timothy, *The 4-Hour Workweek*, New York: Crown Publishing Group, 2009, p. 21.
[88] I highly recommend Garrett Gunderson's myth-busting finance book, *Killing Sacred Cows*, to anyone interested in exploring this subject further (Austin, TX: Greenleaf Book Group, 2008).
[89] Ferriss, *supra* note 87, p. 252.
[90] *Ibid.*, p. 243.
[91] Piedmont, CA: Lawyers' Wellbeing, Inc., 2010.
[92] Ferriss, *supra* note 87, p. 321.
[93] Levit and Linder, *supra* note 84, p. 242.
[94] *Ibid.*, p. 23.
[95] Furlong, Jordan, *Ready for the future? Your survival kit survey results*, Law 21, www.law21.ca/2013/08/ready-for-the-future-your-survival-kit-survey-results/.
[96] Levit and Linder, *supra* note 84, p. 237.
[97] *Ibid.*, p. 67.

To book Andy Clark for a wellness workshop or other speaking
engagement at your law firm, bar association,
or law school, send an email to:
andy@wellnesslawyer.com

To find out more about the Lifebook for Lawyers program
or about Quality of Life Enhancement Coaching, please visit:

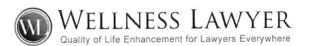

WELLNESS LAWYER
Quality of Life Enhancement for Lawyers Everywhere

www.wellnesslawyer.com